Senior Fitness Test Manual

Roberta E. Rikli, PhD
C. Jessie Jones, PhD

California State University, Fullerton

Human Kinetics

Library of Congress Cataloging-in-Publication Data

Rikli, Roberta E.
    Senior fitness test manual / Roberta E. Rikli, C. Jessie Jones.
        p. cm.
    Includes bibliographical references and index.
    ISBN 0-7360-3356-4
        1. Physical fitness for the aged--Testing--Handbooks, manuals, etc.   2. Exercise for the
    aged--Testing--Handbooks, manuals, etc.   3. Aged--Health and hygiene--Handbooks,
    manuals, etc.   I. Jones, C. Jessie.   II. Title.

    RA781 .R54 2000
    613.7'0446'0287--dc21
                                                                        00-050575

ISBN: 0-7360-3356-4

Acquisitions Editor: Judy Patterson Wright, PhD; **Special Projects Editor:** Anne Cole; **Copyeditor:** Patsy Fortney; **Proofreader:** Jim Burns; **Indexer:** Marie Rizzo; **Permission Managers:** Courtney Astle and Heather Munson; **Graphic Designer:** Stuart Cartwright; **Graphic Artist:** Kathleen Boudreau-Fuoss; **Photo Manager:** Clark Brooks; **Cover Designer:** Keith Blomberg; **Photographer (cover):** Tom Roberts; **Photographer (interior):** Robert A. Peterson © Secure Horizons, except where otherwise noted. Photos on pages 1, 11, 19 (bottom), and 25 provided by the authors. Photos on pages 21 (top), 22 (bottom), and 57 by Tom Roberts. **Art Manager:** Craig Newsom; **Illustrators:** Sharon Smith and John Hatton; **Printer:** United Graphics

Printed in the United States of America   10 9 8 7 6 5 4 3 2 1

Human Kinetics
Web site: www.humankinetics.com

United States: Human Kinetics, P.O. Box 5076, Champaign, IL 61825-5076
800-747-4457
e-mail: humank@hkusa.com

Canada: Human Kinetics, 475 Devonshire Road Unit 100, Windsor, ON N8Y 2L5
800-465-7301 (in Canada only)
e-mail: hkcan@mnsi.net

Europe: Human Kinetics, P.O. Box IW14, Leeds LS16 6TR, United Kingdom
+44 (0) 113 278 1708
e-mail: humank@hkeurope.com

Australia: Human Kinetics, 57A Price Avenue, Lower Mitcham, South Australia 5062
08 8277 1555
e-mail: liahka@senet.com.au

New Zealand: Human Kinetics, P.O. Box 105-231, Auckland Central
09-523-3462
e-mail: hkp@ihug.co.nz

This book is dedicated to our favorite seniors,
our parents—Alfred, Edith, and Florence,
with love and gratitude
for being such positive role models
for successful aging.

Contents

PREFACE

The Senior Fitness Test described in this manual was developed out of a need for a simple, easy-to-use battery of tests to assess physical fitness in older adults. Although physical fitness traditionally has been associated more with younger age groups than with older people, it is most crucial during the later (senior) years. Maintaining adequate strength, endurance, and agility is critical whether our later-life interests are in playing golf, climbing mountains, or performing simple everyday tasks such as climbing stairs or getting out of a chair or bathtub without assistance. In fact, studies suggest that much of the physical frailty commonly associated with aging could be reduced if we paid more attention to our physical activity and fitness as we age, and especially if any evolving weaknesses could be detected and treated early on.

Over the years, however, most tests for assessing physical fitness have been designed for younger people and are not appropriate for older adults. Examples are the FITNESSGRAM developed by the Cooper Institute for Aerobics Research for school-age children (Cooper Institute for Aerobics Research, 1999) and the YMCA Fitness Test Battery (Golding, Myers, & Sinning, 1989), which has 10-year age group norms for adults up to age 65, but not beyond. So far, any tests targeted for older adults have lacked one or more critical components of fitness and/or have been limited in their ability to provide continuous-scale measures across a wide range of functional ability levels, particularly within the field (nonlaboratory) setting.

The lack of a suitable fitness test battery for adults over the age of 60 or 65 quickly became apparent to us as we began developing an on-campus senior fitness program several years ago at the Ruby Gerontology Center at California State University, Fullerton. Obviously, assessments needed to be an important part of this multipurpose program, which was to provide exercise programs for older adults as well as opportunities for research on aging and for educational training for students. We began the process of developing, validating, and norming a new test (the Senior Fitness Test) to meet our needs—that is, one that covered the major components of fitness for older adults (lower- and upper-body strength, aerobic endurance, lower- and upper-body flexibility, and agility/balance), and one that was capable of measuring older people across wide ranges of ages and ability levels. The Senior Fitness Test (SFT) was developed and normed as part of the LifeSpan Project conducted at California State University, Fullerton.[1]

The SFT described in this manual provides a simple, economical method for assessing mobility-related fitness parameters in older adults ages 60 to 90+.

---

[1]The LifeSpan Project, conducted by the authors Drs. Jessie Jones and Roberta Rikli, was made possible in part through the external funding and support of PacifiCare/Secure Horizons, a large health maintenance organization with corporate headquarters in Santa Ana, California. The two-stage project, spanning approximately six years from 1994 to 2000, consisted of developing and validating the test items for the Senior Fitness Test, and conducting and analyzing the results from a nationwide study to establish performance norms and standards for older adults. In the earlier stages of this project, the Senior Fitness Test was sometimes referred to as the LifeSpan Assessments and/or the Fullerton Functional Fitness Test.

Specifically, the test measures the physical attributes (i.e., strength, endurance, flexibility, agility, and balance) needed to perform everyday activities in later life. In addition to being easy to administer and score, the test is safe and enjoyable for older adults, meets scientific standards for reliability and validity, and has accompanying performance standards based on over 7,000 men and women, ages 60 to 94.

An especially important part of the SFT are its normative standards, reported in percentile tables, which make it possible to compare individual scores on each test item with those of other people of the same age and gender. The SFT also has criterion standards (reference points) that indicate the threshold scores on the test items that are associated with the loss of functional mobility and with being at risk for the loss of physical independence in later years.

Another valuable characteristic of the SFT is its ability to discriminate between exercising and nonexercising older adults. Data from our national study indicated that those who were physically active (participated in physical exercise equivalent to at least 30 minutes of brisk walking at least three times a week) scored much better on all test items than did inactive or low-active individuals. In fact, the study provided evidence suggesting that at least half of the usual decline associated with aging might be prevented through regular exercise, or, put another way, that sedentary older people experience twice the amount of physical decline as their more active counterparts.

The SFT is appropriate for use by health and fitness professionals looking to obtain information about the physical status of older adults either for research purposes or for practical application. The test's minimal requirements with respect to equipment, space, and technical expertise make it feasible for use in common clinical and community settings, as well as in the home environment. Also, the test is safe to administer to most older adults without physician approval. The test's multiple uses include providing research data for studies on aging and exercise, assisting health practitioners in identifying weaknesses that may be the cause of mobility problems, and helping fitness and rehabilitation specialists plan appropriate exercise programs for their clients and evaluate their progress over time. With the aid of a partner, the SFT also is suitable for self-administration. However, this manual does not address the procedures and precautions needed for individual use. We are in the process of preparing a separate publication on fitness testing and exercise programs especially for the lay audience.

Although the test battery and its various components have been described previously in various scientific publications (Dugas, 1996; James, 1999; Johnston, 1999; Jones, Rikli, & Beam, 1999; Jones, Rikli, Max, & Noffal, 1998; Rikli & Jones, 1998; Rikli & Jones, 1999a; Rikli & Jones, 1999b), the outpouring of requests for more user-friendly materials convinced us of the need for this additional resource. In the short time since the test was published and presented at several conferences and workshops, we have had hundreds of requests from researchers, health practitioners, and fitness program leaders for additional information and materials. In addition, stories about the test and its use in various programs already have appeared in well over 100 popular press magazines and newspapers such as the *Los Angeles Times*, the *Washington Post*, the *Wall Street Journal*, and *Family Circle* magazine, to name just a few. We also are aware that the SFT is being used in several countries outside the United States including Australia, Brazil, Canada, China, France, Japan, Norway, Portugal, Spain, and South Africa. Clearly, the Senior Fitness Test appears to address an important need in the health/fitness field— that of providing a valid and user-friendly means of evaluating physical ability in the growing population of older adults. As physical activity/fitness programs are rapidly emerging in senior centers and retirement complexes throughout the world, program leaders appear to be crying out for ways of evaluating the status of their clients and of tracking progress within their programs.

The content of the various chapters in this test manual is discussed in the following section. Also available for use with the *Senior Fitness Test Manual* is an accompanying *Senior Fitness Test Video,* which provides visual demonstrations and detailed instructions for administering each of the test items, and *Senior Fitness Test Software*, which can be used to enter and analyze test scores and to provide attractive personalized reports, as well as group statistics showing program outcomes.

ACKNOWLEDGMENTS

The Senior Fitness Test was developed through the cooperative effort of many individuals and organizations. First, we want to express our deep appreciation to the hundreds of people in the local communities surrounding California State University, Fullerton who participated in the numerous background studies for this project—especially the test coordinators and participants at the Ruby Gerontology Center, Leisure World, Morningside Retirement Center, Fullerton and Arcadia Senior Centers, and from the San Diego Adult Education Program. Their participation played a critical role as we refined the test items to meet scientific standards.

Our sincere gratitude also is extended to the hundreds of site supervisors, test coordinators, and volunteer technicians for their effort, dedication, and attention to detail during our national study to establish test norms. In addition, our heartfelt thanks to the over 7,000 older adults throughout the United States who participated in the testing and helped set the standards for the rest of the nation.

Special recognition also goes to our project sponsors, PacifiCare/Secure Horizons for their interest in supporting research designed to enhance the aging process and for their ongoing assistance throughout the various planning and promotional stages of this six-year project. Certainly, a project of this size and duration would not have been possible without their generous financial backing.

We also are especially grateful to our local advisory panel members for their insight and valuable contributions during the test development phase of the project. Members, all of whom are exercise specialists in Southern California, included: William "Bill" Beam, Scott Duncan, Diane Edwards, Laura Gladwin, Blanche Lamar, Charlene Schade, and Greg Welch. In addition, an especially rewarding part of the project was the opportunity to interact with the noted group of distinguished professors, researchers, program directors, and practitioners who served on our national advisory panel. Their expert review of our test development procedures had a significant impact on the quality of the Senior Fitness Test. National advisory panel members (with their affiliations at the time of service) were as follows:

David M. Buchner, MD, MPH
Department of Health Services and Department of Medicine
University of Washington

Wojtek Chodzko-Zajko, PhD
Editor, Journal of Aging and Physical Activity
Kent State University

Janie Clark, MS
President, American Senior Fitness Association
New Smyrna Beach, FL

Loretta DiPietro, PhD
Department of Epidemiology and Public Health
Yale University School of Medicine

Robert Dustman, PhD
Director, Neuropsychology Research
V.A. Medical Center, Salt Lake City

William J. Evans, PhD
Director, Noll Physiological Research Center
Pennsylvania State University

Lawrence A. Golding, PhD
Editor, ACSM Health and Fitness Journal
University of Nevada, Las Vegas

Sheldon Greenfield, MD
Tufts University School of Medicine
Boston, MA

Jack M. Guralnik, MD, PhD
National Institute on Aging
Bethesda, MD

William J. Haskell, PhD
Professor of Medicine
Stanford University

Vivian Heyward, PhD
Professor, Exercise Science
University of New Mexico

Karl Knoph, EdD
President, Fitness Educators of Older Adults Association
Sunnyvale, CA

Jan Montague, MS
Director, Maple Knoll Village Wellness Center
Cincinnati, OH

James R. Morrow, Jr., PhD
Chair of Kinesiology, Health Promotion, and Recreation
University of North Texas

Debra J. Rose, PhD
Director, Motor Behavior Laboratory
Oregon State University

Kay Van Norman, MS
Program Director, Young at Heart
Montana State University

Shelley Whitlatch, MS
Tucson Medical Center Fitness Center
Tucson, AZ

Our sincere appreciation also goes to a special group of experts at Human Kinetics who assisted with the development and publication of the test manual and other related materials. Thank you to Rainer Martens for his vision and direction with respect to the new and exciting *Active Seniors* program, to Judy Wright and Anne Cole for their warm support and valuable assistance in preparing the manuscript, and to Doug Fink and Ernie Noa for their patience and expertise in developing the supportive video and software materials.

And last, but not least, we want to recognize the many faculty, staff, and students at California State University at Fullerton who, over the six-year period of the project, provided assistance and support in so many ways. Finally, it is our hope that the efforts of this "cast of thousands" will be rewarded by the realization that they have contributed in a significant way to an increased fitness awareness and improved quality of life for many current and future older adults.

CREDITS

Figure 2.1 Reprinted, by permission, from R. Rikli & C. Jessie Jones, 1999, "Development and validation of a functional fitness test for community-residing older adults," *Journal of Aging and Physical Activity* 7 (2): 129-161.

Figure 2.2 Reprinted, by permission, from R. Rikli & C. Jessie Jones, 1999, "Development and validation of a functional fitness test for community-residing older adults," *Journal of Aging and Physical Activity* 7 (2): 129-161.

Table 3.1 Adapted, by permission, from R. Rikli & C. Jessie Jones, 1999, "Development and validation of a functional fitness test for community-residing older adults," *Journal of Aging and Physical Activity* 7 (2): 129-161.

Table 3.2 Reprinted, by permission, from R. Rikli & C. Jessie Jones, 1999, "Development and validation of a functional fitness test for community-residing older adults," *Journal of Aging and Physical Activity* 7 (2): 129-161.

Table 3.3 Reprinted, by permission, from R. Rikli and & C. Jessie Jones, 1999, "Development and validation of a functional fitness test for community-residing older adults," *Journal of Aging and Physical Activity* 7 (2): 129-161.

Table 3.4 Reprinted, by permission, from R. Rikli & C. Jessie Jones, 1999, "Development and validation of a functional fitness test for community-residing older adults," *Journal of Aging and Physical Activity* 7 (2): 129-161.

Table 3.5 Reprinted, by permission, from R. Rikli & C. Jessie Jones, 1999, " Functional fitness normative scores for community-residing older adults, ages 60-94," *Journal of Aging and Physical Activity* 7 (2): 162-181.

Figure 3.1a-g Reprinted, by permission, from R. Rikli & C. Jessie Jones, 1999, "Functional fitness normative scores for community-residing older adults, ages 60-94," *Journal of Aging and Physical Activity* 7 (2): 162-181.

Table 5.1 Adapted, by permission, from R. Rikli & C. Jessie Jones, 1999, "Functional fitness normative scores for community-residing older adults, ages 60-94," *Journal of Aging and Physical Activity* 7 (2): 162-181.

Table 5.6 Reprinted, by permission, from G. Borg, 1998, *Borg's Perceived Exertion and Pain Scales* (Champaign, IL: Human Kinetics). The RPE scale occurs on page 47.

How to Use This Manual

This manual presents the information needed to understand the purpose of the Senior Fitness Test (SFT), tells how it was scientifically validated, and explains the procedures for administering the test and interpreting and using the test scores. For a full understanding of the test rationale and procedures, we encourage you to read all of the chapters in the order presented. Realizing, however, that some users may have a greater interest in some portions of the material than in others, we will summarize the main content of each of the chapters.

Chapters 1 and 2 provide the background information for the test and a brief overview of the test's content. Specifically, chapter 1 introduces the test and explains why fitness is just as important, if not more so, for older people as for younger people. The unique features of the SFT, along with suggested ways of using the test are also discussed.

Chapter 2 establishes the conceptual background for the test by explaining how it relates to traditional theories and models describing physical decline in later years. You will see that the test can be used to assess the major physiological components of functional capacity so that emerging physical weaknesses can be detected and treated before they cause serious functional limitations. Included in the chapter is a discussion of the physical parameters that are important for functional mobility (e.g., strength, endurance, flexibility, agility, balance, and body composition) and a list of the criteria used in selecting test items to assess each of these parameters. The overriding goal in developing the test was to select test protocols that meet acceptable scientific standards, but at the same time are economical and easy to administer in the community (nonlaboratory) setting. At the end of chapter 2 you will find a brief overview of each of the test items in the SFT battery.

Chapter 3 contains the scientific documentation for the test's validity, reliability, and performance standards. Our preestablished ground rules for including a test item as part of the SFT battery were that it had to meet the criteria for at least two of three types of validity (i.e., content, criterion, or construct) and have a test-retest reliability of .80 or greater. Also described in this chapter is the nationwide study of over 7,000 independent-living older adults (ages 60 to 94) that provided the data for both norm-referenced and criterion-referenced performance standards. Normative standards provide a basis for comparing an individual's scores to those of others of the same age and gender. Criterion scores suggest the minimum physical ability needed to perform common everyday functions.

Whereas chapters 1 through 3 provide the rationale and scientific documentation for the SFT, chapters 4 and 5 contain the essential "how-to" instructions for test users—how to get ready to administer the tests, how to give the tests, and how to interpret and use the test results.

Included in chapter 4 is a list of procedures and issues that need to be addressed prior to test day, along with sample instruction sheets, forms, and equipment lists to use as you plan for the test. Also included are instructions for warming up the participants on test day and descriptions of the official testing and scoring protocols for each of the SFT items. For those planning to administer the test to classes or groups of individuals, the Guidelines for Group Testing section at the end of the chapter should be especially useful. Included are suggestions for test station setup, group organization and management, and information on selecting and training volunteers to help with testing.

Chapter 5 explains how to interpret the test results and how to use the information to motivate participants to increase their activity level and improve their performance. Included are various performance tables and charts that can help people see how they scored compared to others of their same age and gender and compared to the threshold scores needed to maintain good functional mobility. Also included in chapter 5 is a discussion of ways you can use test results to help your clients set goals and plan effective programs to improve their physical condition. Although a complete discussion of exercise programming for older adults is beyond the scope of this book, we do provide a brief overview of exercise options and activities, as well as a list of additional recommended resources.

The appendixes in the back of the book contain sample forms, tables, and charts presented in copy-ready form, ready to be reproduced and used in your programs. Additionally, appendix N contains a list of other resources that you may find helpful in planning exercise programs for older adults. Finally, you can use the conversion charts in appendix O to convert measurements found in this book from English to metric units.

1

Fitness Testing in Later Years

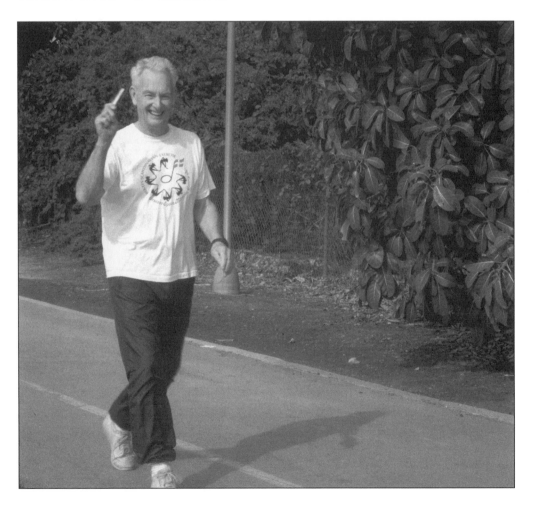

Recognizing Unique Needs of Older Adults

Although physical fitness traditionally has been thought of more as the concern of young people than that of older people, this attitude is changing rapidly. As average life expectancy is increasing, we realize that our ability to enjoy a mobile, active, and independent lifestyle well into the later years will depend to a large degree on how well we maintain our personal fitness level. Whereas health promotion and the avoidance of lifestyle diseases (heart disease, obesity, diabetes, etc.) are the major goals of most youth fitness tests, for older adults whose chronic health status generally has already been established, the focus tends to shift from disease prevention to functional mobility—the ability to continue to do the things one wants and needs to do to stay strong, active, and independent.

The Senior Fitness Test (SFT) described in this manual is a battery of test items that measures the physical capacity of older adults to perform normal everyday activities. The test is considered a functional fitness test as opposed to a health-related fitness test because of its purpose of assessing the physical characteristics needed for functional mobility in later years. Specifically, functional fitness is defined as *having the physical capacity to perform normal everyday activities safely and independently without undue fatigue.* As we age, we want to have the strength, endurance, flexibility, and mobility to remain active and independent so that we can take care of our own personal and household needs; do our own shopping; or participate in active social, recreational, and sport activities, if that's our choice. The SFT is for use by professionals in the fields of health, fitness, and aging who need an economical, easy-to-use assessment tool for measuring older adult fitness in the clinical or community setting. The test was designed to assess independent-living older adults, ages 60 to 90+, across a wide range of ability levels, from the borderline frail to the highly fit.

Chapter 1 overviews fitness testing relative to the unique needs of older adults and introduces the SFT. Specific topics include the following:

- Importance of fitness (and fitness testing) in later years
- Rationale for developing the SFT
- Unique qualities of the SFT
- Uses of the SFT

IMPORTANCE OF FITNESS (AND FITNESS TESTING) IN LATER YEARS

Most of us would agree that quality of life in later years depends to a large degree on being able to do the things we want to do, without pain, for as long as possible. As we are living longer, it is becoming increasingly important to pay attention to our physical condition. Ironically, the numerous technological advances in recent years have had mixed benefits for people relative to quantity and quality of life. Whereas medical technology has contributed to a longer life expectancy, computer/automation technology is resulting in increasingly sedentary lifestyles and an increased risk for chronic health and mobility problems. Statistics suggest that in the United States the health care cost associated with technology-induced inactivity is now approaching $1 trillion per year (Booth, Gordon, Carlson, & Hamilton, 2000). Very few careers or household activities these days provide enough energy expenditure to meet people's physical activity needs. Pushing a button to open the garage door, rolling a trash can out to the curb, or driving through an automated car wash, for example, contribute little to our physical strength, health, and functional mobility.

The surgeon general's 1996 report on physical activity and health provides an excellent overview of the relationship between sedentary lifestyles and the onset of a number of chronic conditions that can lead to frailty and disability in later years (U.S. Department of Health and Human Services, 1996). Further, the recent *Healthy People 2000* review tells us that although life expectancy rates are up and Americans are living longer, more people over the age of 70 are having difficulty performing critical everyday functions such as dressing and bathing (U.S. Department of Health and Human Services, 1999). Unfortunately, it appears that as life expectancy for Americans continues to increase, so too does the possibility of living more years with major physical limitations. We know that many older adults, often due to their sedentary lifestyles, are functioning dangerously close to their maximum ability level during normal activities of daily living. Climbing stairs or getting out of a chair, for example, often require near maximum efforts for older people who are not very physically active. Any further decline or small physical setback could easily cause them to move from independent to disabled status in which assistance is needed for daily activities.

The good news, though, is that much of the usual age-related decline in physical ability is preventable and even reversible through proper attention to our fitness levels and physical activity. Especially important is the early detection of physical weaknesses and appropriate changes in physical activity habits. Until recently, however, most tests to evaluate physical performance were developed either for young people (resulting in tests that are inappropriate, unsafe, or too difficult to complete for many older adults) or for the more frail elderly to determine the amount of care or assistance needed with activities of daily living. Tests that are appropriate for frail older individuals are too easy and not sufficiently challenging to evaluate fitness in healthier, higher functioning older adults (Buchner, Guralnik, & Cress, 1995; Rikli & Jones, 1997; Spirduso, 1995). The SFT, therefore, was developed specifically to evaluate and monitor the physical status of the large population of nonfrail older adults so that evolving weaknesses might be identified and treated before resulting in overt limitations in functional behavior.

> *"The benefits of regular exercise and physical activity contribute to a more healthy, independent lifestyle for seniors, greatly improving their functional capacity and quality of life."*
>
> **—ACSM Position Stand**
> **(American College of Sports Medicine, 1998a)**

RATIONALE FOR DEVELOPING THE SFT

With the surging growth of the older population, finding ways to extend people's active life expectancies and reduce their disabilities have become the goals of government agencies, gerontology researchers, and health practitioners throughout the world. Physical frailty in later years is costly both in terms of the resources spent on medical care and the diminished quality of life for individuals.

Statistics indicate that Americans spend an average of 11.7 years with chronic disabilities that limit their activities of daily living (U.S. Department of Health and Human Services, 1990). Recent figures show that it costs the United States $26 billion a year to care for people who have lost their independence, and these figures are expected to increase drastically as the size of the older population continues to grow (Alliance for Aging Research, 1999). The annual health care cost per person jumps from $4,800 to $36,000 as an older adult progresses from independent to dependent status, with even higher costs incurred when a person has to be institutionalized with full-time care. Some experts believe that disability among older Americans will overwhelm the nation's health care resources and "will drive the cost of health care in this country" for the next 50 years unless ways can be found to reduce or delay frailty and the loss of independence in later years (Alliance for Aging Research).

Although a number of conditions (mental, visual, etc.) can rob people of their independence, problems with physical mobility rank at the top of the list (U.S. Department of Housing and Urban Development, 1999). Luckily, studies suggest that much of the age-related loss in physical function could be prevented or at least reduced with an increased emphasis on lifelong fitness. Also, we know that improvements are possible at any age, even for many of those with chronic health conditions (Kaplan, Strawbridge, Camacho, & Cohen, 1993; Lacroix, Guralnik, Berkman, Wallace, & Satterfield, 1993; Stewart et al., 1994). Research clearly shows that it is never too late to improve one's physical fitness and functional ability; even people in their 90s have experienced dramatic benefits from beginning a physical exercise program (Fiatarone et al.,1990).

In the past, due to the lack of available fitness tests for older adults, health professionals have been limited in their ability to evaluate clients and make recommendations based on objective data. Instead, program leaders generally had to rely on their own subjective judgment in evaluating older people's physical condition and in planning exercise programs. The SFT was developed to address the need for improved ways of assessing fitness in older adults. Specifically, it was designed to assess the functional capacity of the large proportion of nonfrail older adults who are still living independently within the community, but because of their declining fitness levels may soon be at risk for losing their functional independence.

As indicated in the physical function continuum presented in figure 1.1, approximately 70% of the older adult population fits into this independent but generally low-fit category. At the high end of the continuum are the approximately 5% of older adults considered to be functioning at a high-fit or elite level, such as those athletic older people who continue to engage in strenuous exercise or perhaps still participate in athletic competitions. At the lower end are those individuals (representing about 25% of the older population) who already have progressed into the physically frail and dependent categories and need assistance with some or all of their activities of daily living. Although the tests can be adapted for use with more frail older adults, the greatest impact could be made by programs focusing on maintaining independence and preventing frailty in the large midsection of the population. Cost savings in health care expenses and in diminished quality of life would be substantial if we could prevent, or at least delay, older adults' progression from the independent to the frail/dependent category.

UNIQUE QUALITIES OF THE SFT

The SFT was designed to assess physical performance in older adults across a wide range of age groups and ability levels. Although a limited number of other tests also have been developed to assess physiological capacity in older adults (Cress et al., 1996; Guralnik, Ferrucci, Simonsick, Salive, & Wallace, 1995; Osness et al., 1996), the SFT has several unique qualities that distinguish it from others.

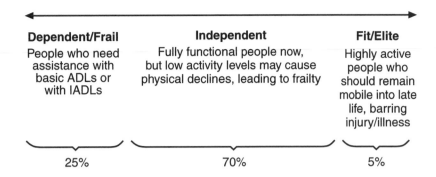

Dependent/Frail
People who need assistance with basic ADLs or with IADLs

Independent
Fully functional people now, but low activity levels may cause physical declines, leading to frailty

Fit/Elite
Highly active people who should remain mobile into late life, barring injury/illness

25% 70% 5%

Figure 1.1 Percentage of older adults (over 70 years of age) classified at various points along a continuum of physical ability (Spirduso, 1995). ADLs refer to the basic activities of daily living such as eating, bathing, and dressing. IADLs are instrumental activities of daily living, that is, activities that are required for independent living such as housework, stair climbing, and shopping. Source: Spirduso, W.W. (1995). *Physical dimensions of aging.* Champaign, IL: Human Kinetics.

- **The SFT is comprehensive.** The test items within the SFT reflect a cross section of the major fitness components associated with independent functioning in later years, whereas other test batteries for older adults focus only on selected aspects of fitness. For example, the EPESE (Established Populations for Epidemiologic Studies of the Elderly) battery includes only tests of lower-body functioning (Guralnik et al., 1994). It measures lower-body strength, balance, and walking speed, but contains no measures reflecting upper-body function. The AAHPERD (American Alliance for Health, Physical Education, Recreation and Dance) test battery, on the other hand, includes a measure of upper-body strength among its test items (the arm curl), but does not address the critical variable of lower-body strength (Osness et al., 1996). The SFT includes measures of upper- and lower-body strength, aerobic endurance, upper- and lower-body flexibility, and agility/dynamic balance. Chapter 2 includes a discussion of relevant fitness parameters for older adults.

- **The SFT provides continuous-scale measures.** Another unique feature of the SFT is that it produces continuous-scale scores on all test items across a broad range of ability levels from the borderline frail to the highly fit. A common limitation in other test batteries is that some items tend to be either too easy or too difficult for a large portion of community-residing older adults, resulting in "ceiling" or "floor" effects in the measurement data (Rikli & Jones, 1997).

A ceiling effect occurs when a test is too easy for much of the population of interest, resulting in a large number of perfect scores. In the large EPESE populations, for example, nearly 50% of those tested received perfect scores (i.e., reached the ceiling or upper limit) on a test of tandem balance, thus eliminating the discrimination ability of that item for half of the participants (Guralnik et al., 1994; Seeman et al., 1994). Conversely, a floor effect occurs when a test is too difficult for the population of interest. Because many older people cannot complete the half-mile distance walk in the AAHPERD test (that is, cannot reach the lower limits of the test), it is said to have a floor effect for some people. Because the score on the half-mile test is the time it takes to complete the test, anyone unable to walk the required distance (an estimated 40% of the older population) will not receive a score (Select Committee on Aging, 1992).

The testing protocols of the SFT, on the other hand, were designed to minimize ceiling and floor effects. The SFT uses a distance-based scoring system, for example, for its walking test (i.e., how far a person can walk in 6 minutes), as opposed to a time-based scoring system (the time it takes to walk a prescribed distance, such as half a mile), thus making it possible for all participants to obtain a score. Scores can be obtained for frail individuals who can walk only a few feet in 6 minutes, as well as for highly fit older adults who can cover several hundred yards within the time period.

- **The SFT is usable in the field setting.** Because the items in the SFT have minimal equipment and space requirements, the entire battery can be administered in most clinical and community (nonlaboratory) settings, as well as in people's homes. Some tests, on the other hand, such as the Continuous-Scale Physical Functional Performance Test (CS-PFP) developed by Cress et al. (1996) have special equipment needs that require them to be performed in a laboratory or other specialized setting. Although the strength of the CS-PFP is that its various test components involve real-life everyday activities such as boarding a bus or transferring laundry from a washer to a dryer, the standardization of these tasks requires that it be administered in very specialized environments with specific types of equipment.

- **The SFT has accompanying performance standards.** Another especially important feature of the SFT is that it has accompanying performance standards for use in evaluating test results. Specifically, the SFT has five-year age group percentile norms for independent-living men and women, ages 60 to 94, on all test items, thus making it possible for individuals to evaluate their scores relative to others of their same age and gender. Data for the norms were obtained in a nationwide study involving over 7,000 older adult volunteers from 267 test sites in 21 different states. The tables and charts presented in chapter 5 indicate the percentile scores for each test item, along with scoring ranges that would be considered above normal, normal, or below normal. In addition, the scores on each test item that were associated with self-reported loss of functional ability by the study participants provide a type of criterion standard or reference point indicating increased risk for losing independence. See chapter 3 for further discussion of the at-risk scoring thresholds.

USES OF THE SFT

The SFT is appropriate for use by health and fitness professionals looking to collect data either for research purposes or for practical application. Specific examples of how the test might be used are discussed here.

- **Conducting research.** Because the SFT has documented reliability and validity, it can be used to provide dependable data in a variety of settings: it can provide baseline scores for longitudinal or prospective studies, posttest measures for evaluating intervention effects, and accurate measures for correlation analyses in cross-sectional studies. Also, because the test does not require extensive equipment, time, space, or technical expertise, it should be especially useful to researchers needing to collect physical performance data within the community (nonlaboratory) setting or even in people's homes. In addition, the continuous-scale scoring ability of the SFT can provide researchers with a richer set of data than would measures that provide only ranked or categorical scores.

- **Evaluating individuals and identifying risk factors.** Taking the SFT can tell individuals whether their physical capacities rank in the above-normal, normal, or below-normal categories compared to others of their same age and gender. Test results can also show people how close they are to the threshold scores that may signify being at risk for losing functional independence. Also, by taking the test on multiple occasions and tracking their scores over time, people can monitor changes in performance. They will know if they are improving or declining—and if declining, whether at a slower or faster rate than that of other people their age. Individual assessment can help to identify specific areas of physical weakness that will need attention if declines leading to loss of function are to be prevented or reduced.

• **Planning programs.** Group or individualized exercise programs designed to improve functional mobility should be based on as much information as possible to maximize program effectiveness and participant safety. The SFT provides information on physical strengths and weaknesses, thus providing the background information needed to develop fitness programs that target the specific needs of individuals or groups. In fact, program leaders who already are using the SFT tell us that the inclusion of testing has added quality and substance to their programs, as well as additional participants.

> *"The Senior Fitness Tests have made all the difference in the world in our programs. Finally, we now have a way of measuring the progress of our clients. The tests are easy to give and people enjoy taking them and seeing how they are doing. In fact, we have built a whole exercise program around these tests—they are so functional and make so much sense."*
>
> **—Maribeth Peniger, Director of the Forever Fit Program (Colorado Springs, Colorado)**

• **Educating and setting goals.** Careful interpretation of the test results to participants can help them better understand how their fitness levels relate to their functional mobility. Poor scores on lower-body flexibility, for example, generally indicates that the hamstring muscle group is not very flexible. Instructors or therapists can explain to their clients that reduced flexibility in the lower body is associated with poor posture, low back pain, problems with walking, and possibly an increased risk of falling. Test results also can provide a meaningful basis for developing an individual's short- and long-term goals. An example of a short-term goal might be to improve performance by 20% by the end of a 12-week program, or perhaps to move from the 25th percentile in one's age group to the 50th percentile. An example of a more long-term goal might be to be able to comfortably walk a full mile without stopping by the following summer—a goal that could be especially relevant to someone who is planning an oversees trip and needs more confidence in his or her ability to keep up with the tour group. Participant goals should always play a major role in planning fitness programs for older individuals. For most people, setting personal goals tends to increase motivation and improve exercise compliance. See chapter 5 for additional information on goal-setting.

• **Evaluating Programs.** Previous research has indicated that exercise leaders rarely conduct physical assessments of their clients (Schroeder, 1995). Increasingly, however, program leaders are being asked to provide evidence of outcome measures to document a program's effectiveness. The following are examples of possible program goals (which in turn can provide outcome measures) for a newly scheduled exercise class. By the end of a 12-week program: (1) At least 75% of the participants will improve their fitness and mobility. (2) The average SFT scores of class participants will improve by 20%. (3) Over 50% of the participants will report feeling better and having more energy for performing everyday activities.

An example of a more global or long-term outcome measure might be evidence showing that over a three-year period exercise participants either improved or maintained their fitness level, compared to nonexercisers who experienced the usual age-related declines in physical ability.

> *"The LifeSpan Project (Senior Fitness Test) has been very helpful to us here in Georgia. The Georgia Division of Aging Services has required that goals and outcome measures be a part of all sponsored programs. We use these tests to provide a measurable way of gauging how clients are progressing in the exercise programs that have been implemented. We have been very excited about these tests and their results."*
>
> **Tena Eddy-Pulley, Director of Fitness Programs,**
> **Center for Positive Aging (Atlanta, Georgia)**

• **Motivating Clients.** Most people are inherently curious about their physical abilities and how they compare with those of others of their same age and gender. The performance tables and charts in chapter 5 make it possible for participants to compare their scores to their peers and to track their physical changes over time. Other participants may be more interested in comparing their scores to specified standards, such as the at-risk threshold scores presented in the performance charts in chapter 5. Still others, especially the more competitive individuals, may be motivated to try to score at the top of the scale in their age groups on all test items. Again, the normative tables provide the information needed for evaluating one's performance compared to others.

• **Improving Public Relations.** The U.S. Department of Health and Human Services has set a national health goal of increasing Americans' number of active years and reducing physical frailty (1999). Test results obtained at regular intervals can be used to evaluate individual progress or to document a program's overall effectiveness relative to such goals. Such results can provide the basis for a press release focusing on a program's success in serving local community needs or in addressing a particular political agenda. Positive media coverage is not only good public relations, but also very helpful in attracting resources for programs and for recruiting additional participants.

SUMMARY

Our personal fitness level is important at any age. As we get older, however, the focus shifts from health promotion to functional mobility. Functional fitness is defined as having the physical capacity to perform normal everyday activities safely and independently without undue fatigue. We developed the SFT to provide a simple, economical method for assessing functional fitness in older adults ages 60 to 90+. The SFT distinguishes itself from other tests in that it

• is comprehensive,

- provides continuous-scale measures,
- is usable in the field setting, and
- has normative performance standards.

Health and fitness professionals will find many uses for the tests, including the following:

- Conducting research
- Evaluating individuals and identifying risk factors
- Planning programs
- Educating and setting goals
- Evaluating programs
- Motivating clients
- Improving public relations

In the next chapter we will describe the procedures used to identify the relevant parameters of functional fitness, as well as the criteria established for selecting the specific test items to assess those parameters. Also included in the chapter will be a brief overview of the test items and their scoring protocols.

2

THE SENIOR FITNESS TEST

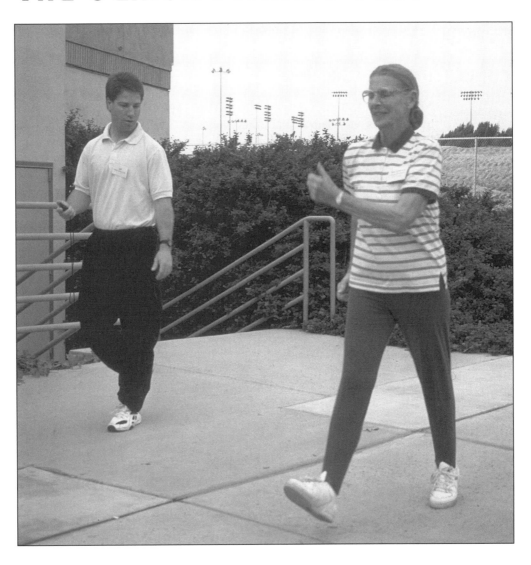

Defining Functional Fitness Parameters

In developing the Senior Fitness Test (SFT) battery it was important to first identify the major fitness parameters associated with functional mobility, and then to select specific test protocols to assess these parameters. To accomplish these tasks we reviewed the literature on factors related to functional mobility, solicited input from a panel of nationally noted experts in the fields of gerontology and exercise relative to the appropriate content for the SFT, and used an advisory board of exercise leaders from our local community to help pilot-test the protocols to determine their clarity and feasibility for use in the field setting.

This chapter contains background information acquired through our review of literature and through feedback and input from our expert advisory panels. Included in the chapter is information on

- the conceptual background for the test development;
- a functional fitness framework illustrating the relationship among fitness parameters, functional behaviors, and activity goals;
- the criteria used in selecting test items to assess each of the fitness parameters; and
- a brief overview of the test items and their scoring protocols.

CONCEPTUAL BACKGROUND

An initial step in developing the SFT was to consider the role of physical activity and fitness within the disability process. The traditional models explaining the disabling process (Nagi, 1965, 1991) describe four main stages in the progression to disability: (1) disease/pathology, (2) physiological impairment, (3) functional limitation, and (4) disability. More specifically, the model (figure 2.1a) suggests that pathology leads to physiological impairment (decline in body systems, i.e., muscular, cardiovascular, neurological, etc.), physiological impairment leads to functional limitations (restrictions in physical behaviors such as rising from a chair, lifting, or climbing stairs), and functional limitation leads to disability (the inability to perform normal daily activities such as bathing oneself, housework, or shopping).

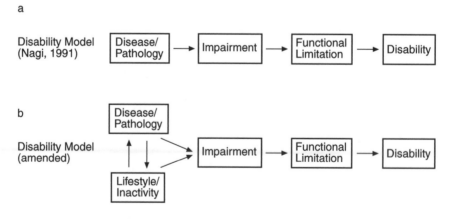

Figure 2.1 *(a)* Nagi's 1991 model of the progression leading to disability and *(b)* an amended version suggesting that an inactive lifestyle can have comparable effects on the disabling process.
Reprinted from Rikli & Jones 1999.

Although traditionally it was thought that all disability originated from disease or pathology, recent evidence suggests that a physically inactive lifestyle also can be a primary cause of frailty in later years especially for people living into their 80s and 90s, and that the model should be amended as shown in figure 2.1b (Chandler & Hadley, 1996; DiPietro, 1996; Morey, Pieper, & Cornoni-Huntley, 1998; Rikli & Jones, 1997). In fact, data suggest that physical inactivity is on a par with chronic disease as a cause of disability, and that increased physical activity is associated with higher levels of functional mobility in people who have chronic health problems as well as in those who are relatively healthy (Kaplan et al., 1993; Lacroix et al., 1993; Seeman et al., 1995; Stewart et al., 1994).

More relevant to the importance of fitness testing, however, is evidence that physical decline, whether due to disease or to disuse, is modifiable through proper assessment and activity intervention. Studies show that increased physical activity, even when begun late in life, results in improved physical fitness (strength, endurance, etc.), as well as in improved functional ability (walking, stair climbing, etc.) (Cress, et al., 1991; Fiatarone et al., 1990; Fiatarone et al., 1994; McCartney, Hicks, Martin, & Webber, 1996; Nichols, Hitzelberger, Sherman, & Patterson, 1995; Pyka, Lindenberger, Charette, & Marcus, 1994; Rikli & Edwards, 1991). In the McCartney et al. study (1996), continuous strength improvements during a two-year exercise program were accompanied by continued improvements in related functions such as walking, stair climbing, and cycling.

Understanding both the contributing causes of physical decline (e.g., disease and inactivity) and the subsequent stages leading to frailty is helpful in planning effective prevention strategies and in designing relevant measurement tools. The SFT was designed specifically to assess performance at the physiological stage (muscular, cardiovascular, etc.) so that performance in these critical supporting parameters might be evaluated and monitored, thus helping to curtail declines that might lead to additional losses, especially losses that progress to the point of affecting everyday functioning.

> *"Over one-third of nursing home admissions are primarily caused by mobility-related problems."*
>
> **U.S. Department of Health and Human Services, 1991**

FUNCTIONAL FITNESS PARAMETERS

In developing the SFT, the functional ability framework described in figure 2.2 provided us with a useful guide in defining functional fitness and in identifying the relevant physical parameters that ought to be included as part of a functional fitness test. Consistent with the disability models described by Nagi and others (Lawrence & Jette, 1996; Nagi, 1991; Rikli & Jones, 1997), and with research on physical activity and fitness in older adults, the framework illustrates the progressive relationship among physical parameters, functional abilities, and activity goals. The common activities in the far right column in figure 2.2 (e.g., taking care of personal needs, household chores, shopping, or traveling) require the ability to perform the functions listed in column 2 (e.g., walking, stair climbing, lifting, and reaching). These functions, in turn, require an adequate reserve in the physical parameters identified in column 1—muscular strength, aerobic endurance, flexibility, and agility/balance—as well as an optimal, or at least manageable, body mass index (relationship of height to weight).

Physical Parameters	Functions	Activity Goals
Muscle strength/ endurance	Walking	Personal care
Aerobic endurance	Stair climbing	Shopping/errands
Flexibility	Standing up from chair	Housework
Motor ability power speed/agility balance	Lifting/reaching	Gardening
Body composition	Bending/kneeling	Sports
	Jogging/running	Traveling

Physical impairment → Functional limitation → Reduced ability/ disability

Figure 2.2 Functional ability framework. Indicates the physiologic parameters associated with functions required for basic and advanced everyday activities.
Reprinted from Rikli & Jones 1999.

Based on the functional fitness framework in figure 2.2, and the supporting research, the following physical parameters were identified as being the relevant components of functional fitness:

- Muscular strength (lower- and upper-body)
- Aerobic endurance
- Flexibility (lower- and upper-body)
- Agility/dynamic balance
- Body mass index

A brief discussion of these parameters and their relevance to functional mobility is presented in the following sections.

Muscular Strength

According to fitness experts, maintaining muscular strength should be the number one fitness concern of older adults (Evans & Rosenberg, 1991; Fiatarone & Evans, 1993; Haskell & Phillips, 1995; Nelson et al., 1994; Pendergast, Fisher, & Calkins, 1993). A decline in muscle strength, which averages about 15% to 20% per decade after the age of 50 (American College of Sports Medicine, 1998a; Shephard, 1997), can have devastating effects on people's ability to perform normal everyday activities. Lower-body strength is needed for activities such as climbing stairs, walking distances, or getting out of a chair or bathtub. Upper-body strength is important for carrying groceries, lifting a suitcase, picking up a grandchild or a pet, and for many other common tasks. Statistics indicate that many older people, due to their declining strength, begin losing their ability to perform these functions fairly early in the aging process. In a nationally-representative sample of over 6,000 community-residing adults over 70, 26% could not climb even one set of stairs without stopping, 31% had difficulty lifting 10 pounds (a bag of groceries), and 36% reported having trouble walking several blocks (Stump, Clark,

Johnson, & Wolinsky, 1997). Although both lower- and upper-body strength impairments are associated with the inability to perform activities of daily living (Fried, Ettinger, Lind, Newman, & Gardin, 1994; Lawrence & Jette, 1996), decreasing lower-body strength is an especially powerful predictor of the onset of disability in later years (Gill, Williams, Richardson, & Tinetti, 1996; Guralnik et al., 1995; Lawrence & Jette, 1996).

Maintaining strength and muscle function is also important because of the role it plays in helping to reduce the risks for falls and fall-related injuries (Bohannon, 1995; Brown, Sinacore, & Host, 1995; Judge, 1993; MacRae, Feltner, & Reinsch, 1994; Tinetti, Speechley, & Ginter, 1988), and because of its positive effect on a number of age-related health conditions. Muscular strength can help reduce bone loss, improve glucose utilization, maintain lean body tissue, and prevent obesity (Evans & Rosenberg, 1991; Haskell & Phillips, 1995).

Although the decline in muscle mass and strength can be attributed to multiple factors such as genetics, disease, and nutrition, the most important variable related to muscle loss in older adults is physical inactivity. Fortunately, research now shows that through increased exercise it is possible for people of any age to regain much of their lost strength and muscle mass, and as a result, experience improved functional mobility (Evans, 1995; Fiatarone et al., 1990; Fiatarone et al., 1994; McCartney et al., 1996). Because of the significance of maintaining muscular strength during aging, its measurement (both lower- and upper-body) is an important aspect of fitness evaluation and program planning for older adults.

Aerobic Endurance

An adequate level of aerobic endurance (the ability to sustain large-muscle activity over time) is necessary to perform many everyday activities such as walking, shopping, sightseeing while on vacation, or participating in recreational or sport activities. How much work our bodies can do and how much energy we have is related to how much oxygen we can take in and use. Although it has been estimated that a $\dot{V}O_2$max (a common measure of oxygen consumption/aerobic capacity) of 15 to 18 ml $\times$ kg^{-1} $\times$ min^{-1} is necessary to maintain independent living status, declines associated with inactive lifestyles often progress below this point prior to age 80 (Paterson, Cunningham, Koual, & Croix, 1999; Shephard, 1997).

Although aerobic capacity tends to decline at the rate of 5% to 15% per decade after the age of 30, resulting in as much as a 50% loss by the age of 70, studies indicated that at least half of this decline could be avoided by being physically active (Hagberg, 1994; Jackson et al., 1995; Jackson et al., 1996). Maintaining an adequate level of aerobic activity has both a direct effect on a person's functional mobility and an indirect effect through its role in helping to reduce the risk for such medical conditions as cardiovascular disease, diabetes, obesity, high blood pressure, and some forms of cancer (U.S. Department of Health and Human Services, 1996).

As was true of muscular strength, research also shows that increased exercise can lead to substantial improvements in aerobic endurance in older adults (American College of Sports Medicine, 1998a). In fact, data now show that endurance exercise training in older adults can lead to the same amount of improvement as that found in young adults (Hagberg et al., 1989; Kohrt et al., 1991). Clearly, aerobic endurance is an important fitness component for older adults.

Flexibility

The importance of flexibility relative to one's fitness level increases with age. Loss of flexibility (i.e., loss of range of motion around a joint) impairs most functions needed for good mobility, including bending, stooping, lifting, reaching, walking, and stair climbing (Badley, Wagstaff, & Wood, 1984; Konczak, Meeuwsen, & Cress, 1992). Maintaining lower-body flexibility, especially in the hip joint and hamstrings, is also important because of its role in preventing low back pain, musculoskeletal injury, gait abnormalities, and in reducing the risk of falling (American College of Sports Medicine, 1995; Grabiner, Koh, Lundin, & Jahnigen, 1993; Kendall, McCreary, & Provance, 1993; Liemohn, Snodgrass, & Sharpe, 1988).

In the upper body (shoulder area), adequate range of motion is needed for a number of specific functions such as combing one's hair, zipping a back zipper, putting on or removing over-the-head garments, removing a wallet from a back pocket, or reaching for a seat belt. Reduced range of motion in the shoulder girdle also can result in pain and postural instability (Magee, 1992) and has been found to cause significant disability in as much as 30% of the healthy adult population over 65 (Chakravarty & Webley, 1993). Both lower- and upper-body flexibility, both of which decline with age but can be improved through exercise (Hubley-Kozey, Wall, & Hogan, 1995; Morey et al., 1991; Rikli & Edwards, 1991), are important aspects of functional fitness for older adults.

Agility/Dynamic Balance

Combined agility (involving speed and coordination) and dynamic balance (maintaining postural stability while moving) is important for a number of common mobility tasks that require quick maneuvering such as getting on and off a bus in a timely manner; moving out of the way to avoid getting hit by a car or other object; or getting up quickly to answer a phone call, go to the bathroom, or tend to something in the kitchen. Also, adequate agility/dynamic balance is needed for safe participation in many recreational games and sports.

Although some might argue that agility and dynamic balance represent two different components of fitness and should be evaluated separately, we are treating them as one composite measure since both must work together for the successful performance of many everyday activities, such as the ones mentioned earlier. Studies indicate that performance on combined agility/dynamic balance tasks is related to gait speed, to other measures of balance, and to a composite index reflecting activities of daily living, and is a predictor of recurrent falling (Podsiadlo & Richardson, 1991; Tinetti, Williams, & Mayewski, 1986). Data from our recent study to establish norms for the SFT indicate that the rate of decline on the agility/dynamic balance task is similar to that of other variables and that physical exercise is an important factor in maintaining agility and balance (Rikli & Jones, 1999b).

Body Mass Index

The composition of a person's body, particularly the ratio of fat to lean tissue, can have a marked impact on one's health and functional mobility. People with excess body fat relative to their muscle mass are not going to be able to function (manage their bodies) as well as people with normal ratios of fat and muscle. Starting around age 30, people typically begin gaining weight at the average rate of one pound per year until about age 50 (for men) or 60 (for women), after which there usually is a weight stabilization for a few years and then a gradual decline in weight. Unfortunately, for most people the weight decline in later years usually is not due to a loss in fat, but to a loss in lean body tissue (muscle mass and bone). Although body mass index (BMI), a weight/height ratio measure, is not a direct reflection of body composition, it is more highly correlated with body weight than with body height and, therefore, has been used for years as a general indication of healthy weight management (Shephard, 1997).

We have recommended that BMI be included as part of the SFT because of the role it plays in maintaining functional mobility. Studies indicate that people who are overweight (typically due to excess body fat) are more likely to be disabled in later years than are people with normal body mass ratings. Similarly, researchers are finding that people with very low BMIs are at increased risk for health and mobility problems, possibly due to an associated loss in muscle mass and/or bone tissue (Galanos, Peiper, Cornoni-Huntley, Bales, & Fillenbaum, 1994; Harris, Kovar, Suzman, Kleinman, & Feldman, 1989; Losonczy et al., 1995).

Body mass index can be determined by multiplying weight in pounds by 703 and dividing by height in inches squared: BMI = $(lbs \times 703)/in^2$. BMI also can be estimated by referring to the BMI Conversion Chart in appendix F. Although it has not been determined what the optimal BMI range is for older adults, values between 19 and 26 are generally considered to be in the healthy range, with BMIs higher or lower associated with increased risk for health and mobility problems (American College of Sports Medicine, 1998b; Evans & Rosenberg, 1991; Galanos et al., 1994; Harris et al., 1989; Losonczy et al., 1995; Shephard, 1997).

In summary, research suggests that the following physiological parameters are especially important in supporting functional mobility in later years: muscular strength (lower- and upper-body), aerobic endurance, flexibility (lower- and upper-body), agility/dynamic balance, and body composition. The importance of these variables relative to the physical health and mobility of older adults has also been documented in a number of major reviews and reports (American College of Sports Medicine, 1997, 1998a; Bouchard, Shephard, & Stephens, 1994; Buchner, 1995; Chandler & Hadley, 1996; Hurley & Hagberg, 1998; Morey et al., 1998; U.S. Department of Health and Human Services, 1996).

After identifying the physiological components to be represented in the battery, the next step was to select specific test protocols that could measure these parameters—protocols that were reliable and valid and would meet other test development goals such as being easy to use in a field (nonlaboratory) setting. Following is a list of the criteria that we established to serve as guidelines in selecting the test items.

TEST SELECTION CRITERIA

In selecting the test items for the SFT, consideration was given to two overriding goals: (1) the development of test protocols that meet acceptable scientific standards with respect to test reliability and validity; and (2) the development of tests that would be easy to administer and feasible for use in common clinical, community, and home settings where the majority of older adult assessment is likely to take place. More specifically, with input from our advisory panels, we established the following criteria to use as guidelines during the test development. It was agreed that all test items should

- Represent a cross section of the major functional fitness components—i.e., key physiologic parameters associated with functional mobility.

- Have acceptable test-retest reliability ($\geq$ .80) (Safrit & Wood, 1995).
- Have acceptable validity, with documentation to support at least two of the following: content, criterion, and/or construct (discriminant) validity. For acceptable criterion validity, correlations between the test item and the criterion measure were to be at least .70, preferably above .80 (Safrit & Wood, 1995). For construct/discriminant validity, relevant group differences were to be significant beyond the .01 level (Baumgartner & Jackson, 1999). Content (logical) validity was to be established through literature review and through the subjective judgment of expert reviewers.
- Reflect usual age-related changes in physical performance.
- Be able to detect physical changes due to training or exercise.
- Be able to assess performance on a continuous scale across a wide range of functional abilities from the low fit/borderline frail to the high fit. The goal was to avoid ceiling and floor effects so that all, or most, participants could receive a score.
- Be easy to administer and score.
- Require minimum equipment and space so they can be administered in typical clinical and community settings, as well as in the home.
- Be safe to perform without medical release for the majority of community-residing older adults.
- Be socially acceptable, meaningful, and motivating to older people.
- Be reasonably quick to administer, with individual testing time requiring no more than 30 to 40 minutes, and with groups of up to 24 people being able to complete the test within a 60- to 90-minute period, using trained volunteer assistants.

Developing test items to meet the previously cited criteria required extensive trial-and-error pilot testing, with the main focus on adapting and refining test protocols to meet the standards for reliability and validity while at the same time assuring minimal requirements with respect to time, equipment, and space. The involvement of the local advisory board members was especially useful during this stage of the test development. We used their programs to conduct pilot tests and to obtain feedback relative to the feasibility of test protocols for use in field settings. Ultimately, the following seven test items and one alternate were selected for inclusion in the SFT.

OVERVIEW OF TEST ITEMS

Following is an overview of each of the test items selected for inclusion in the SFT. The purpose of each item is given, along with a brief description of the test protocol. Additional rationale for each test item is presented in chapter 3 as part of the discussion on test validity. Detailed descriptions of the test protocols can be found in chapter 4.

■ ■ CHAIR STAND TEST

Purpose:

To assess lower-body strength needed for numerous tasks such as climbing stairs; walking; and getting out of a chair, tub, or car. Increased ability in performing this exercise may reduce the chance of falling.

Description:

Number of full stands from a seated position that can be completed in 30 seconds with arms folded across chest.

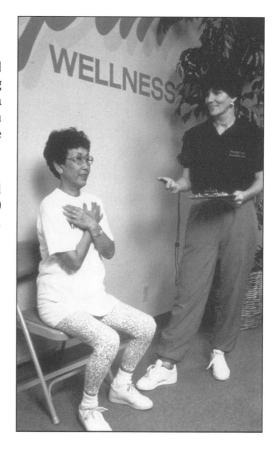

■ ■ ARM CURL TEST

Purpose:

To assess upper-body strength needed for performing household and other activities involving lifting and carrying things such as groceries, suitcases, and grandchildren.

Description:

Number of biceps curls that can be completed in 30 seconds holding a hand weight—5 lbs (2.27 kg) for women, 8 lbs (3.63 kg) for men.

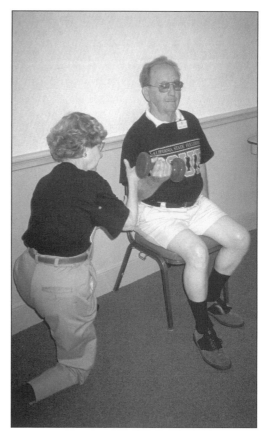

▪▪ 6-MINUTE WALK TEST

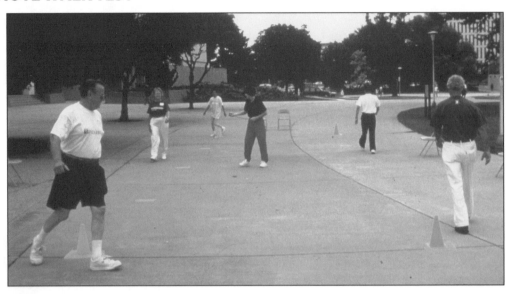

Purpose:

To assess aerobic endurance—important for walking distances, climbing stairs, shopping, sightseeing while on vacation, etc.

Description:

Number of yards (meters) that can be walked in 6 minutes around a 50-yard (45.72-meter) course.

▪▪ 2-MINUTE STEP TEST

Purpose:

Alternate aerobic endurance test for use when time, space limitations, or weather prohibits giving the 6-minute walk test.

Description:

Number of full steps completed in 2 minutes, raising each knee to a point midway between the patella (kneecap) and iliac crest (top hip bone). The score is the number of times the right knee reaches the required height.

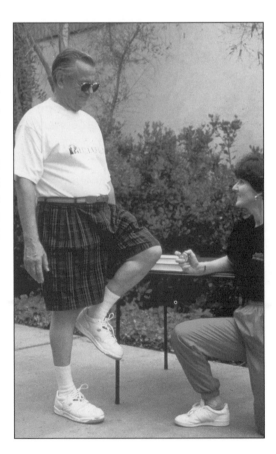

■ ■ CHAIR SIT-AND-REACH TEST

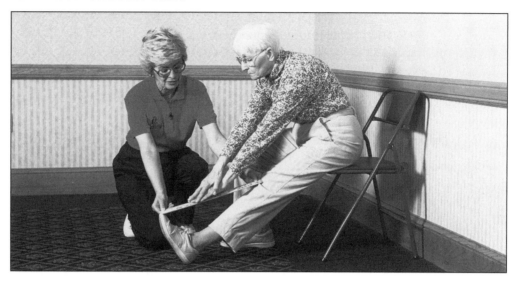

Purpose:

To assess lower-body flexibility, which is important for good posture, normal gait patterns, and various mobility tasks such as getting in and out of a bathtub or car.

Description:

From a sitting position at the front of a chair, with leg extended and hands reaching toward toes, the number of inches (centimeters) (plus or minus) between the extended fingers and the tip of the toe.

■ ■ BACK SCRATCH TEST

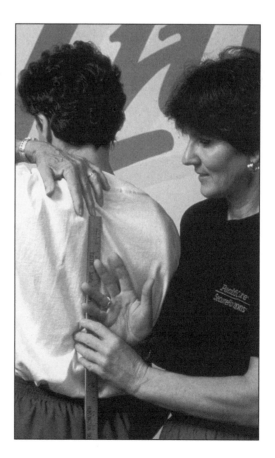

Purpose:

To assess upper-body (shoulder) flexibility, which is important in tasks such as combing one's hair, putting on overhead garments, and reaching for a seat belt.

Description:

With one hand reaching over the shoulder and one up the middle of the back, the number of inches (centimeters) between the extended middle fingers (plus or minus).

■ ■ 8-FOOT UP-AND-GO TEST

Purpose:

To assess the agility/dynamic balance important in tasks that require quick maneuvering such as getting off a bus in time, getting up to attend to something in the kitchen, going to the bathroom, or answering the phone.

Description:

Number of seconds required to get up from a seated position, walk 8 feet (2.44 meters), turn, and return to seated position.

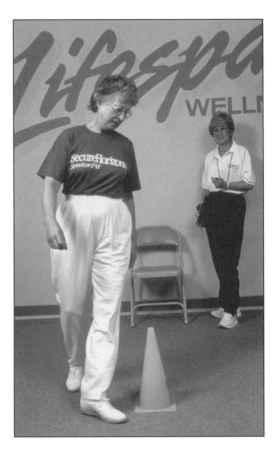

■ ■ HEIGHT AND WEIGHT

Purpose:

To assess body weight relative to body height, because of the importance of weight management for functional mobility.

Description:

Involves measuring height and weight, then using a conversion table to determine body mass index.

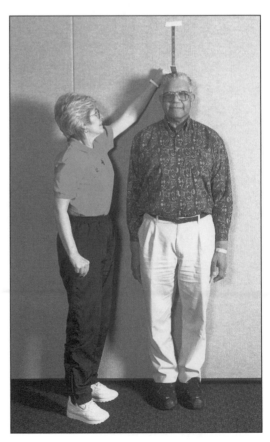

SUMMARY

In developing the SFT, we first identified the fitness parameters needed for functional mobility, then selected test items to assess these parameters. According to disability models, physical impairment (loss of strength, endurance, etc.) resulting from either pathology or disuse is the initial stage in the progression to disability. Physical impairment, in turn, leads to functional limitation (restriction in physical behaviors such as rising from a chair or climbing stairs), which eventually can lead to disability (loss of ability to take care of oneself).

Identifying the key physiological attributes associated with functional mobility is important in developing physical assessments and in planning exercise prevention/rehabilitation programs. Based on a literature review and feedback by expert judges, the following were identified as being key physiological parameters related to functional mobility in older adults:

- Muscular strength (lower- and upper-body)
- Aerobic endurance
- Flexibility (lower- and upper-body)
- Agility/dynamic balance
- Body mass index

After identifying the general components of functional fitness, the next step was to develop testing protocols to assess each fitness parameter. To meet the goals of the SFT, it was important that the test items

- be reliable and valid;
- be sensitive enough to detect expected changes in performance due to aging or to exercise intervention;
- be able to assess a wide range of performance levels, from borderline frail to highly fit;
- be easy to administer and score and have minimal requirements with respect to equipment, time, space, and training; and
- be socially acceptable and motivating to older people.

Following considerable trial-and-error pilot testing to develop protocols to meet the previously cited criteria, the following test items were selected for inclusion in the SFT battery:

- Chair stand test (lower-body strength)
- Arm curl test (upper-body strength)
- 6-minute walk test (aerobic endurance)
- 2-minute step test (an alternate measure of aerobic endurance)
- Chair sit-and-reach test (lower-body flexibility)
- Back scratch test (upper-body flexibility)
- 8-foot up-and-go test (agility/dynamic balance)
- Height and weight (body composition)

In the next chapter we will describe the procedures followed in assuring that these test items meet the standards of quality required for an effective test. Specifically, we will discuss the procedures used for establishing test validity and reliability and for developing norm-referenced and criterion-referenced performance standards for the SFT.

3

TEST VALIDITY, RELIABILITY, AND PERFORMANCE STANDARDS

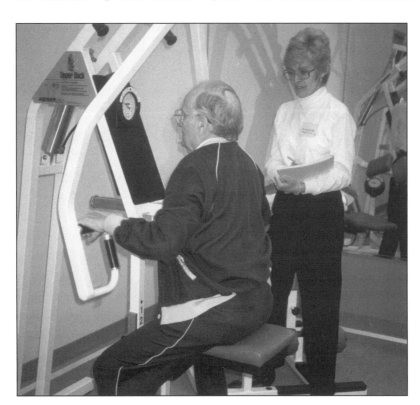

Identifying Relevant Fitness Measures for Older Adults

For a test to be of value, whether for research purposes or for practical application, it must be valid and reliable (American Psychological Association, 1985). A valid test is one that measures what it is intended to measure. A test developed to measure bicep strength, for example, would be considered valid if it can be shown to measure the strength of the bicep muscles. A reliable test is one that results in consistent, dependable, and repeatable test scores free of measurement error. A test is considered reliable if it produces the same scores when given on different occasions, assuming no change in the ability level of the test takers.

According to American Psychological Association (APA) guidelines, published tests also should have some type of performance standards or scales that can help users interpret test results. Common types of performance standards are norm-referenced and criterion-referenced. Norm-referenced standards (norms) are used to judge a person's performance in relation to others of a clearly defined group, such as older adult men, for example. Criterion-referenced standards are those that reflect a level of performance that is needed to achieve a particular goal, or that provide "cut-points" for placing people into categories, such as being healthy versus being at risk for disease, or being functionally capable versus functionally dependent. In developing the SFT, it was our goal to establish normative performance standards for men and women ages 60 to 90+, and to begin to identify criterion standards or minimum fitness thresholds associated with maintaining functional independence.

This chapter describes the processes involved in establishing the validity and reliability of the SFT[1], as well as the procedures used for developing performance standards. The topics include the following:

- Validity
    - Types of validity evidence
    - Validity evidence for the SFT items
- Reliability
    - Procedures for estimating reliability
    - Reliability of SFT items
- Performance standards
    - Norm-referenced standards
    - Criterion-referenced standards

VALIDITY

The single most important characteristic of any test is its validity. Because a valid test is one that measures what it is intended to measure, its validity must always be determined relative to its purpose. For example, if a test item's purpose is to measure lower-body strength, then one way of evaluating its validity is to compare scores from that test with scores on an already proven test of lower-body strength. A high correlation between the two sets of scores would indicate good test validity relative to the criterion measure. However, if the test's purpose is also to be able to detect differences between people who exercise and those who don't, then further evidence of the test's validity would be data show-

[1] In earlier publications and materials that described the development of the SFT, it has been referred to as the LifeSpan Assessments and the Fullerton Functional Fitness Test.

ing that exercising people score higher on the test than do nonexercising people. Ideally, tests should be validated using as many sources of evidence as possible.

Types of Validity Evidence

The major sources of evidence for establishing test validity are grouped into three categories: content-related, criterion-related, and construct-related (American Psychological Association, 1985).

Content-Related Validity

Content validity (or logical validity, as it often is called when referring to physical performance measures) is the degree to which a test reflects a defined universe or domain of content, such as functional fitness in the case of the SFT. According to the APA standards, support for content validity can come from a data-based literature review showing the relevance of the various test components, as well as from the subjective judgment of experts in the field. The content relevance (or logical validity) of the fitness categories included in the SFT was addressed in chapter 2 in the section on Functional Fitness Parameters. In that section, we documented the importance of various fitness parameters relative to maintaining functional mobility in later years, specifically, lower-body strength, upper-body strength, aerobic endurance, lower-body flexibility, upper-body flexibility, agility/dynamic balance, and body composition.

The scientific advisory panel provided further support of the content validity of the SFT parameters, and of the selection of specific test items to assess the parameters. The advisory panel, consisting of 16 nationally noted authorities in the fields of gerontology and exercise science, provided feedback and consultation during key phases of the test development. Panel members' names and affiliations are listed in the acknowledgments section in the front of this book. We solicited information from panel members on both a formal and informal basis. On some occasions all panel members responded in writing to a specific set of questions about the appropriateness of the test rationale and test content. On other occasions, as needed, we asked individual panel members to answer specific questions based on their respective areas of expertise. Throughout the test development, we used feedback from the panel to make adjustments in test content and protocols.

Criterion-Related Validity

Criterion-related validity is the degree to which a test correlates with a criterion measure, that is, a measure already known to be valid (American Psychological Association, 1985). Criterion validity generally is estimated by calculating the correlation coefficient (Pearson's r) between scores on the test being validated with scores on the comparison measure of performance. Evidence supporting the criterion validity of the SFT items comes from a combination of previously published data on measures similar to the SFT items and from new studies designed specifically to look at each SFT item relative to a criterion measure, whenever a criterion measure could be identified. The validation studies and the specific criterion measures used are discussed in the section on Validity Evidence for SFT Items.

Construct-Related Validity

Construct validity, or discriminant validity as it sometimes is called, is the degree to which a test measures a particular construct of interest (American Psychological

Association, 1985). A construct is an attribute that exists in theory but cannot be observed directly such as intelligence, personality, or in this case, functional fitness (strength, endurance, etc.). The process of establishing construct validity typically begins with the development of a conceptual framework that explains the meaning and relevance of the construct and continues until studies are able to confirm expected predictions or inferences about the construct (American Psychological Association, 1985). An expected inference about the construct of strength, for example, would be that exercisers would have a higher level of strength than nonexercisers. Studies confirming this prediction would provide evidence of the construct validity (discrimination ability) of the particular strength measure involved. This method of establishing construct validity is referred to as the group differences method (Safrit & Wood, 1995). Differences between groups are tested for significance using appropriate statistical procedures, either a *t* test (for two groups) or analysis of variance (for more than two groups).

Support for the construct validity of the SFT items comes from material discussed in the sections on Conceptual Background and Functional Fitness Parameters in chapter 2 and from new validation studies specifically designed to test the ability of the SFT to detect expected fitness differences in older adults of different ages and activity levels. These studies were conducted with 190 male and female residents (mean age = 76.2 years) from a retirement housing complex. Scores on each of the test items were analyzed to determine the test's ability to detect expected performance differences (declines) over three decades—the 60s, 70s, and 80s— as well as expected differences in people with high and low levels of physical activity.

Physical activity was assessed through self-report, using a simple questionnaire that asked about exercise frequency and intensity level. High-active people were those who indicated that they participated in moderate physical activity (strenuous enough to cause a noticeable increase in breathing, heart rate, and perspiration) at least three times a week. Low-active people were those who were active less than three times a week or not at all. Simple questionnaires, such as the one used in this study, provide a reliable and valid way of classifying individuals into high- and low-activity categories (Ainsworth, Montoye, & Leon, 1994; Paffenbarger, Blair, Lee, & Hyde, 1993).

All participants in the study were functionally independent and ambulatory without the use of an assistive device (cane or walker) and were free of medical conditions that would prohibit their performance on the tests. Participants were primarily Caucasian (90%), female (80%), and from above-average socioeconomic backgrounds. See Rikli and Jones (1999a) for additional details. Study results are discussed under each of the separate test items in the following section.

Validity Evidence for SFT Items

Presented here is a brief discussion of the purpose and background of each of the SFT items, followed by the evidence supporting the validity of each item. A full description of each of the SFT items is presented in chapter 4. The validity evidence presented is based on both previously published data, which provide support for the content validity, and sometimes the criterion validity, of each test item, and on new data from validation studies conducted as part of the SFT project.

Chair Stand Test

The purpose of the chair stand test is to assess lower-body strength, an important aspect of fitness in older adults because of its role in common everyday activities such as stair climbing; walking; maintaining balance; and getting out of a chair, bathtub, or car. The test involves counting the number of times, within a 30-second time period, that a person can come to a full stand from a seated position with arms folded across the chest.

Background. The 30-second chair stand test is a modification of other versions of chair stand tests that involve recording the time it takes to complete a specified number of stands such as 10 stands (Csuka & McCarty, 1985) or 5 stands (Guralnik et al., 1994). The reason for changing the protocol from measuring the time it takes to complete a specific number of stands to counting the number of stands that can be completed in a specific amount of time (30 seconds) was to improve the scoring effectiveness (discriminant ability) of the test. In the 5- and 10-stand versions of the test, if people are unable to complete the required number of stands, which many cannot, then they do not receive a score. In one large-scale study, for example, involving several thousand community-residing older adults, over 20% of the participants could not complete even 5 stands (Guralnik et al., 1994). Using a standardized time protocol (such as 30 seconds) instead of a standardized number protocol (such as 5 or 10) makes it possible for everyone to receive a score, even though the score would be zero for someone who could not complete even one chair stand within the 30-second period. See the chair stand test protocol in chapter 4 for complete details.

Validity Evidence. Past studies show that chair-stand performance, a common method of assessing the lower-body strength of older adults in the field setting, correlates reasonably well with laboratory measures of lower-body strength (e.g., Cybex II knee extensor and knee flexor strength) and with other indicators of interest such as walking speed, stair-climbing ability, and balance (Bohannon, 1995; Csuka & McCarty, 1985). Chair-stand performance also has been found to be effective in detecting normal age-related declines (Csuka & McCarty), in discriminating between fallers and nonfallers (MacRae, Lacourse, & Moldavon, 1992), and in detecting the effects of physical training in older adults (McMurdo & Rennie, 1993). Studies also show that chair-stand performance is associated with the risk of falling (Alexander, Schultz, & Warwick, 1991; Tinetti, Speechley, & Ginter, 1988).

Specifically, to test the criterion validity of the chair stand test used in the SFT, test scores were compared to leg press strength as measured by a Keiser double leg press machine. The leg press, a multiple-joint exercise involving hip extension, knee extension, and ankle plantar flexion, is an especially relevant criterion measure of lower-body strength for older people. This measure reflects the kind of strength needed for many everyday activities such as rising from a chair, getting in and out of a tub or a car, or stooping to pick something up from the floor (Judge, 1993). Leg press was measured using a 1-RM (repetition maximum) protocol that had previously been determined to have high test-retest reliability in older adults (Rikli, Jones, Beam, Duncan, & Lamar, 1996). The moderately high correlation between chair stand test scores and leg press scores ($r = .78$ for men and .71 for women; see table 3.1) provides criterion-related evidence of the test's validity as a measure of lower-body strength (Jones, Rikli, & Beam, 1999).

In support of the construct (discriminant) validity of the chair stand test, study results showed the test's ability to detect expected performance declines across each decade from the 60s to the 80s. Exact means and standard deviations are given in table 3.2. Also, as expected, scores from the chair stand test were significantly higher for participants with high levels of physical activity than for participants with low levels. As indicated in table 3.3, high-active participants completed an average of 13.3 stands in 30 seconds compared to only 10.8 by low-active participants.

Table 3.1 Criterion Validity of Senior Fitness Test Items

Test item	Criterion measure	Men & women r (n)	Men r (n)	Women r (n)	References
Chair stand	1-RM leg press	.77 (89)	.78 (40)	.71 (49)	Jones, Rikli, and Beam, 1999
Arm curl	Combined 1-RM biceps, chest, and upper back		.84 (33)	.79 (35)	James, 1999
6-min walk	Time on treadmill to 85% max heart rate	.78 (37)	.82 (17)	.71 (20)	Rikli & Jones, 1998
2-min step	1-mile walk time Time on treadmill to 85% max heart rate	.73 (24) .74 (25)			Dugas, 1996 Johnston, 1999
Chair sit-and-reach	Hamstring flexibility (American Academy of Orthopaedic Surgeons)	.83 (80)	.76 (32)	.81 (48)	Jones et al., 1998
Back scratch	No single criterion available	Considered to be best overall measure of shoulder flexibility			Gross, Fetto, & Rosen, 1996 Starkey & Ryan, 1996
8-ft up-and-go	No single criterion available	Considered to be a good measure of combined physiologic attributes (power, speed, agility, and balance) encountered in common behaviors			Podsiadlo & Richardson, 1991 Tinetti et al., 1986

Adapted from Rikli and Jones 1999.

Table 3.2   SFT Means and Standard Deviations for 60-, 70-, and 80-Year-Olds

Test item	60-69 yrs	70-79 yrs	80-89 yrs	$p^\dagger$
	($n = 32$) (91% female)	($n = 96$) (84% female)	($n = 62$) (81% female)	
Chair stand (# in 30 sec)	14.0 (2.4)	12.9 (3.0)	11.9 (3.6)	.013*
Arm curl (# in 30 sec)	19.8 (4.1)	18.2 (3.9)	16.5 (4.1)	.007*
6-min walk (total yd)	677.8 (95.0)	621.0 (82.4)	550.1 (86.7)	.0001*
2-min step (# in 2 min)	100.4 (9.0)	92.6 (16.0)	83.5 (22.6)	.0001*
Chair sit-and-reach (in. from toe)	−0.4 (5.4)	−0.4 (6.2)	−3.3 (6.0)	.018**
Back scratch (in. from middle fingers)	1.0 (2.0)	−0.4 (3.0)	−1.8 (4.4)	.0009*
8-ft up-and-go (seconds)	5.2 (0.6)	6.1 (1.2)	7.1 (2.0)	.0001*

Mean ages for the 60-, 70-, and 80-year-old groups were 65.9 (3.5), 75.1 (2.9), and 83.3 (3.0), respectively.

† Significance level of ANOVA F ratios.

* ANOVA and post hoc analyses revealed that all three age groups differed significantly.

** The 80-year-olds were significantly different from the 60- and 70-year olds, but the 60- and 70-year-olds did not differ from each other.

Reprinted from Rikli and Jones 1999.

Further support for the construct validity of the chair stand test was provided in a recent replication study that was designed to provide an independent analysis of the reliability and validity of the SFT items using a separate sample of independent-living older men and women (Miotto, Chodzko-Zajko, Reich, & Supler, 1999). Of the 69 participants in this study, 42 were described as physically active (mean age = 67.9) and 37 as sedentary (mean age = 69.4). Results showed that the chair stand test again was successful in detecting expected differences between active and inactive subjects, with the active group averaging 17 stands in 30 seconds compared to only 13 for the sedentary group. The overall higher scores for participants in the Miotto et al. study may be due to the fact that they were somewhat younger (in their late 60s) compared to those in the Jones et al. (1999) study, in which mean ages were 75.6 for high-active and 77.7 for low-active participants.

Arm Curl Test

The arm curl test is included in the SFT as a general measure of upper-body strength, which is needed to perform many everyday activities such as housework and yard work, and for lifting and carrying things such as groceries, suitcases, grandchildren, and pets. The test involves counting the number of times a

Table 3.3   SFT Means and Standard Deviations of High-Active and Low-Active Participants

Test item	High-Active	Low-Active	p (t ratios)
	(n = 136) (88% female)	(n = 47) (84% female)	
Chair stand (# in 30 sec)	13.3 (2.8)	10.8 (3.6)	.0001
Arm curl (# in 30 sec)	18.7 (4.0)	15.5 (3.7)	.0001
6-min walk (total yd)	647.6 (81.5)	513.2 (77.9)	.0001
2-min step (# in 2 min)	95.8 (15.7)	72.8 (18.4)	.0001
Chair sit-and-reach (in. from toe)	−0.6 (6.0)	−3.8 (6.6)	.007
Back scratch (in. from middle fingers)	−0.3 (3.4)	−2.1 (3.8)	.005
8-ft up-and-go (seconds)	6.0 (1.3)	7.1 (2.1)	.0001

High-active participants were those who, according to self-report, were regular participants (at least three times a week) for at least one year in physical exercise or activity that was strenuous enough to cause a noticeable increase in heart rate, breathing, or perspiration. Low-active participants were new enrollees in exercise classes who had not participated in regular exercise for at least five years. Mean ages: high-active = 75.6 yrs (SD = 6.6); low-active = 77.7 yrs (SD = 6.9).

Reprinted from Rikli and Jones 1999.

person can curl a hand weight, 5 lbs (2.27 kg) for women and 8 lbs (3.63 kg) for men, through the full range of motion in 30 seconds.

Background. The arm curl test in the SFT is similar to the arm curl test described in the AAHPERD functional fitness test (Osness et al., 1996) with two exceptions: (1) a change in the prescribed weight for women from a 4-lb (1.8-kg) to a 5-lb (2.27-kg) weight, and (2) a change in arm position during the curl-up phase of the movement. The 5-lb weight for women was selected for the SFT because upper-body strength in women tends to be about 60% of that of men (Sperling, 1980), thus improving the representation of the female/male weight ratio (5 lbs for women versus 8 lbs for men). The change in arm position from the handshake grip used in the AAHPERD test to a palm-up protocol during flexion in the SFT test was to more effectively engage the muscles of the upper arm and the biceps tendon relative to muscle action. In the SFT arm curl test, the participant starts the test holding the weight in the handshake position at full extension (arm down at side), then supinates during flexion so that the palm of the hand faces the biceps at full flexion. See the arm curl test procedure in chapter 4 for complete details.

Validity Evidence. At the time the SFT was being developed, a review of the literature revealed little research addressing the validity of the arm (biceps) curl as an indicator of upper-body strength in older adults. The only reference found for the arm curl (using hand weights) indicated that it had a .82 correlation with

Cybex arm curl scores. However, these data were from an unpublished study involving only seven subjects (Osness et al., 1996). Therefore, to assess the potential of the arm curl test as an indicator of overall upper-body strength, we designed a study to compare arm curl test scores with scores on a composite criterion measure of upper-body strength—a combined measure that included 1-RM biceps, chest press, and seated rowing scores as measured on weight resistance machines (James, 1999). The results of this study involving 68 older adults (33 men, mean age = 74; and 35 women, mean age = 71) indicated that the correlation between the arm curl test scores and the composite strength measures were .84 for men and .79 for women (see table 3.1). These moderately high correlations provide support for the criterion validity of the arm curl test as a measure of overall upper-body strength. Previous studies indicated that the protocol followed on the 1-RM strength tests was highly reliable for older adults (James, 1999; Rikli & Jones, 1999a).

As with the chair stand test, the arm curl test also was successful in detecting expected age-related declines in strength from the 60s to the 70s to the 80s and in discriminating between regular and nonregular exercisers (Rikli & Jones, 1999a), thus supporting the construct (discriminant) validity of the test. The mean scores for these comparison groups are given in tables 3.2 and 3.3. As indicated, there was a consistent decrease in the average number of curls performed across the three decades (decreasing from 19.8 to 18.2 to 16.5), and scores were lower, as expected, for low-active individuals (15.5 curls) than for high-active individuals (18.7 curls).

Further evidence of the discrimination ability of the arm curl test was provided in the subsequent replication study by Miotto et al. (1999) in which physically active participants scored significantly better than sedentary individuals. The average number of arm curls completed in 30 seconds was 23 for the active group compared to 19 for the sedentary group (Miotto et al., 1999). Again, the higher scores in the Miotto et al. study is probably due to the fact that their participants were younger (average ages were in the late 60s) than those in the SFT studies, in which the average ages were 75.6 and 77.7 years for the high-active and low-active groups, respectively.

Grip strength, measured by a grip dynamometer, is another common field-test measure of upper-body strength in younger people. However, this was not considered an acceptable option for older adults due to the discomfort associated with performing this test, especially for the numerous older people with arthritis in their hands. Results of a pilot study conducted at Fullerton indicated that participants with arthritis were much less bothered performing the arm curl test than the grip strength test.

6-Minute Walk Test

The purpose of the 6-minute walk test is to assess aerobic endurance, defined as the capacity to perform large-muscle activity over an extended time. Aerobic endurance is needed to perform a variety of activities including stair climbing, walking, shopping, sightseeing while on vacation, and participating in active sport and recreational activities. The test involves walking continuously around a 50-yard (45.72-meter) course, covering as much distance as possible in 6 minutes.

Background. The rationale for standardizing the time (6 minutes) in the SFT instead of a specified distance, such as half a mile or a mile as is common in other distance walking tests (Kline, et al., 1987; Osness et al., 1996), was to improve the scoring effectiveness (discrimination ability) of the test. On a timed test, such as the 6-minute walk, scores can be obtained for individuals of all ability levels—

from the borderline frail who can walk only a few feet in 6 minutes, to the highly fit who can cover several hundred yards in the time allowed. Because reports show that a considerable number of community-residing older adults (at least one third of those over 70) have difficulty walking even a few blocks (Select Committee on Aging, 1992; Stump, Clark, Johnson, & Wolinsky, 1997), tests with prescribed distances (such as half a mile or a mile) would be prohibitive to many elderly people.

Validity Evidence. Past studies generally show that distance walking tests of various types (half-mile, 12-minute, and 1-mile) are reasonably good indicators of aerobic endurance in both young adults (Cooper, 1968; Disch, Frankiewicz, & Jackson, 1975; Kline et al., 1987) and high-functioning older adults (Bravo, et al., 1994; Fenstermaker, Plowman, & Looney, 1992; Warren, Dotson, Nieman, & Butterworth, 1993). Also, studies show that walking tests of shorter durations, such as 5-minute or 6-minute walking tests, correlate well with cardiorespiratory endurance in older people with various medical conditions (Bittner et al., 1993; Guyatt et al., 1985a; Peloquin, Gauthier, Bravo, Lacombe, & Billiard, 1998). However, before the development of the SFT, the 6-minute walk test had not been validated on relatively healthy, independent-living older adults.

To further test the criterion validity of the 6-minute walk as a measure of aerobic (cardiovascular) endurance, we designed a study that compared the 6-minute walk test scores of 77 independent-living older men and women (mean age = 73 years) with submaximal treadmill walking performance using a modified, previously validated Balke protocol (American College of Sports Medicine, 1991). Scores collected during the Balke graded exercise test represented total time on the treadmill before reaching 85% of predicted maximum heart rate. Results revealed an overall correlation of .78 between 6-minute walk test scores and scores on the treadmill test, indicating moderately good criterion-related validity (Rikli & Jones, 1998). The correlations for men and women separately were .82 and .71, respectively. See table 3.1.

Submaximal physical performance (as opposed to a measure of maximal oxygen consumption) was selected as the criterion measure in the study because of its greater relevance to older adult functioning. Maximal oxygen consumption measures have been found to have questionable relevance to the demands of everyday activities for older adults and do not correlate well with measures of daily functioning (Bittner et al., 1993; Guyatt et al., 1985b; Steele, 1996).

As with most other SFT measures, the 6-minute walk test was successful in detecting expected performance differences across age groups (60s, 70s, and 80s) and in people with different levels of physical activity (high versus low), thus providing construct-related evidence of the test's validity (see tables 3.2 and 3.3). Additional construct-related validity evidence was provided in the same study when it was found that 6-minute walk test scores, as expected, were significantly higher for people with self-reported high levels of functional ability compared to those who reported difficulty with many common everyday activities. Functional ability in this study was assessed using a 12-item self-report scale indicating a person's ability to perform functions ranging from personal care chores such as dressing and bathing to higher-level functions such as heavy housework and strenuous exercise (Rikli & Jones, 1998).

2-Minute Step Test

The 2-minute step test is included in the SFT battery as an alternate measure of aerobic endurance when space limitations (or sometimes weather conditions) prohibit use of the 6-minute walk test. The 2-minute step test protocol involves determining the number of times in two minutes that a person can step in place raising the knees to a height halfway between the patella (kneecap) and iliac crest (front hip bone). See the 2-minute step test diagram in chapter 4.

Background. The 2-minute step test might be considered a self-paced version of several previously published tests such as the Harvard Step Test (Brouha, 1943), the Ohio State Step Test (Cotten, 1971), and the Queens College Step Test (McArdle, Katch, Pechar, Jacobson, & Ruck, 1972), all of which require a specified stepping cadence. Pilot testing during the early stages of the SFT development clearly showed that many older adults cannot or will not maintain a prescribed stepping cadence, thus making these tests inappropriate for this population. Originally, our idea for the self-paced, step-in-place test came from a similar measure developed in Canada as part of the Post 50 "3-S" Physical Performance Test (Bell, Hoshizaki, & Collins, 1983). A review of the literature, however, revealed no validation studies on self-paced step tests.

Validity Evidence. Scores on most previously published step tests, such as those mentioned earlier that involve stepping at a preset cadence onto a bench of a prescribed height, tend to be moderately well correlated with recognized measures of aerobic capacity. A correlation of .75, for example, was found between $\dot{V}O_2$max scores and step test scores for college women using the Queens College Step Test (McArdle et al., 1972). On a sample of college men, a correlation of .84 was found between Ohio State Step Test scores and maximum aerobic capacity values obtained from a Balke treadmill protocol (Cotten, 1971). Although numerous additional reports could be cited that look at the validity of step tests with young people, no studies were found involving older participants.

In developing the SFT, we conducted a series of studies at Fullerton to compare 2-minute step test scores with other published measures of aerobic endurance. Dugas (1996) found a moderate correlation ($r = .73$) between 2-minute step test scores and Rockport 1-mile walk scores in 24 older men and women (mean age = 69.6). In another study involving 25 older men and women (mean age = 70.8), a similar correlation ($r = .74$) was found between 2-minute step test scores and treadmill performance (Johnston, 1999). Treadmill performance represented time on the treadmill until the participant reached 85% of his or her predicted maximum heart rate, using a modified Balke graded exercise protocol (American College of Sports Medicine, 1991). As indicated in tables 3.2 and 3.3, the 2-minute step test was able to detect expected performance declines across each decade from the 60s to the 80s and was able to discriminate successfully between exercisers and nonexercisers.

It also was interesting to note that data collected on the rate of perceived exertion (RPE) during the 2-minute step test were fairly comparable to those collected from the same participants during the 6-minute walk test, suggesting that the two aerobic endurance tests are similar with respect to exercise intensity. On a scale of 6 to 20 (Borg, 1998) the average RPE reported during the step test was 13.9 compared to 13.6 during the 6-minute walk test. These RPE scores represent a degree of exertion that is between "somewhat hard" (13.0 on the scale) and "hard" (15.0 on the RPE scale).

Chair Sit-and-Reach Test

The purpose of the chair sit-and-reach test is to assess lower-body flexibility, particularly hamstring flexibility, which is important for good posture and for mobility tasks such as walking, stair climbing, and for getting in and out of a car or bathtub. Lower-body flexibility also helps prevent low back pain and musculoskeletal injuries, and reduces the risk of falling. The test involves sitting at the front edge of a stable chair, with one leg extended and the other foot flat on the floor. With hands on top of each other and arms outstretched, the object is to reach as far forward as possible toward the toes. The score is the number of inches (centimeters), either plus or minus, between the tips of the middle fingers and the toes.

Background. The chair sit-and-reach test in the SFT was adapted from earlier versions of floor sit-and-reach tests that have appeared in numerous test batteries including the YMCA battery (Golding, Myers, & Sinning, 1989), FITNESSGRAM (Cooper Institute for Aerobics Research, 1999), and the AAHPERD Functional Fitness Test for Adults Over 60 (Osness et al., 1996). Most versions of the sit-and-reach test involve sitting on the floor with both legs extended and reaching as far forward as possible toward (or past) the toes. An exception is the FITNESSGRAM back-saver sit-and-reach, which involves sitting on the floor but extending only one leg at a time while the other is bent.

We chose to move from a floor to a chair protocol for the SFT flexibility test because many older adults have medical conditions or functional limitations (obesity, low back pain, lower-body weakness, hip and knee replacements, severely reduced flexibility, etc.) that make it difficult or impossible for them to get down and up from a floor position. In our pilot studies we also found that some older people, probably due to a combination of weak abdominal muscles and tight hamstrings, could not hold a sitting position on a flat surface, particularly with both legs extended.

In the chair sit-and-reach test, as in the back-saver version of the sit-and-reach test recommended in the FITNESSGRAM (Cooper Institute for Aerobics Research, 1999), only one leg is extended at a time while the other is bent with the foot flat on the floor. The rationale for keeping one leg straight and one bent during the testing, as opposed to both legs straight, is based on evidence showing that the simultaneous stretching of both hamstrings causes excessive posterior disc compression, thereby increasing the risk of back injury during the testing (Cailliet, 1988).

Validity Evidence. Past studies indicate that sit-and-reach tests, in general, have at least moderate criterion-related validity relative to established measures of hamstring flexibility, with r values ranging from .61 to .89 (Jackson & Baker, 1986; Jackson & Langford, 1989; Patterson, Wiksten, Ray, Flanders, & Sanphy, 1996). However, to our knowledge, no prior studies have been published investigating the potential effectiveness of a chair version of the sit-and-reach as a method of assessing lower-body (hamstring) flexibility. Therefore, to assess the criterion-related validity of the newly developed chair sit-and-reach test, we conducted a study to compare its scores with goniometer-measured hamstring flexibility, a common gold standard measure of lower-body flexibility (American Academy of Orthopaedic Surgeons, 1966). As indicated in the published report of the study (Jones, Rikli, Max, & Noffal, 1998) and also in table 3.1, the correlation between chair sit-and-reach test scores and the goniometer-measured criterion was .81 for the 48 female participants (mean age = 74.0 years) and .76 for the 32 males (mean age = 74.5). In fact, data from the study also showed that the scores from the chair version of the sit-and-reach test were better correlated to hamstring flexibility in older people than were scores from the floor sit-and-reach test, even for people who had no trouble getting down and up from the floor position (Jones et al., 1998).

Relative to the discrimination ability (construct validity) of the chair sit-and-reach test, the data in table 3.2 indicate that scores were only partially successful in detecting expected differences among the various age groups in the study. The 80-year-olds, as expected, had significantly lower flexibility scores than 60- or

70-year-olds, but there was no difference between the 60- and the 70-year-old groups. Further study will be needed to determine whether the lack of observed change in flexibility between 60- and 70-year-olds is due to the inability of the chair sit-and-reach test to detect such change or whether, in fact, it is due to a true lack of change in flexibility during this period. The chair sit-and-reach test was successful, however, in discriminating between high-active and low-active participants. As seen in table 3.3, high-active participants, on the average, could reach within .6 inches (1.52 centimeters) of their toes, whereas the average score for low-active people was a negative 3.8 inches (–9.65 centimeters).

Back Scratch Test

The purpose of the back scratch test is to assess upper-body flexibility, particularly shoulder flexibility, which is important in performing common tasks such as combing one's hair, zipping a dress, putting on an over-the-head garment, or reaching for a seat belt. Reduced range of motion in the shoulder also can result in pain and increased chance of injury and disability in later years (Chakravarty & Webley, 1993; Magee, 1992). The test involves reaching one hand over the shoulder and down the back as far as possible and the other hand around the waist and up the middle of the back as far as possible, trying to bring the fingers of both hands together. The score is the number of inches (centimeters), either plus or minus, between the extended middle fingers.

Background. The back scratch test is a modified version of the Apley scratch test that has been used for years by therapists and orthopedic physicians as a quick way of evaluating overall shoulder range of motion (Gross, Fetto, & Rosen, 1996; Hoppenfeld, 1976; Magee, 1992; Starkey & Ryan, 1996). The Apley protocol, which involves reaching behind the head with one hand and behind the back with the other hand toward a specified anatomical point on the opposite scapula, was revised slightly to involve simply trying to touch the middle two fingers together behind the back. The change in assessment protocol was to provide a simpler and more quantifiable method of measuring shoulder range of motion in the field setting.

Validity Evidence. Although no single criterion measure exists for the Apley test, it is considered by experts in the field to be a valid assessment of overall shoulder range of motion (Gross et al., 1996; Hoppenfeld, 1976; Starkey & Ryan, 1996). The motion of reaching behind the head and over the shoulder reflects shoulder flexion, abduction, and external rotation. The behind-the-back position involves shoulder extension, adduction, and internal rotation.

Similar versions of this test are included in other published test batteries such as FITNESSGRAM (Cooper Institute for Aerobics Research, 1999) and the Brockport Physical Fitness Test (Winnick & Short, 1999), but no studies to date have been published describing the criterion validity of these measures. The shoulder stretch test in the FITNESSGRAM involves the same motions as the back scratch in the SFT, although the scoring systems are different. In the FITNESSGRAM, scores are either yes (fingers can touch behind the back) or no (fingers cannot touch), whereas the back scratch test in the SFT involves measuring the distance between the two middle fingers, thus providing a continuous-scale scoring system. The modified Apley test in the Brockport battery involves evaluating only one arm at a time as the person attempts to reach behind the head toward the opposite scapula. Data from an unpublished pilot study indicate some support for the relationship between the modified Apley scores and functional ability in a group of individuals with cerebral palsy (Winnick & Short, 1999).

The logical (content) validity of the Apley and related shoulder stretch tests has been fairly well established based on the extent of its use by therapists and physicians as a tool in evaluating shoulder range of motion (Gross et al., 1996; Hoppenfeld, 1976; Starkey & Ryan, 1996). Studies involving the SFT back scratch test provide support for the construct (discrimination) validity of the test. The back scratch test was able to detect expected declines in shoulder flexibility across age groups (60s, 70s, and 80s), as well as expected differences between participants with high and low activity levels (Rikli & Jones, 1999a). The mean scores for each of these comparison groups can be found in tables 3.2 and 3.3. In a subsequent study, Miotto et al. (1999) found that shoulder flexibility measured using the SFT back scratch test was only slightly worse for sedentary older adults than for a group of active seniors, differences that were not statistically significant. Although more studies are needed to verify the criterion-related and construct-related validity of the back scratch test, the evidence supporting its logic (content validity) as an overall measure of shoulder flexibility appears strong.

8-Foot Up-and-Go Test

The purpose of the 8-foot up-and-go test is to assess agility and dynamic balance, attributes that are needed for a number of functions such as getting up and maneuvering quickly enough to get off a bus in time, attend to something in the kitchen, go to the bathroom, or answer the phone or the door in a timely manner. The test involves getting up from a seated position and walking as quickly as possible around a cone (or similar marker) that is 8 feet (2.44 meters) away and returning to the seated position.

Background. The 8-foot up-and-go test is a modified version of a previously published 3-meter "timed up-and-go" protocol (Podsiadlo & Richardson, 1991). The main purpose in changing the distance from 3 meters (9.84 feet) to 8 feet was to increase the feasibility of administering this test in areas with limited space, particularly in the home setting. In our pilot studies we found that although it often was difficult to find the needed space in many areas to administer the 3-meter test (which must include room for turning around the cone), we almost always could find space to set up an 8-foot version of the test. Fortunately, our reliability studies showed that little to no accuracy was lost in shortening the distance.

Validity Evidence. Although there is no one gold standard criterion measure to compare performance on the 8-foot up-and-go test, it has been found to be significantly related to the Berg Balance Scale ($r = .81$), to gait speed ($r = .61$), and to the Barthel Index of ADLs ($r = .78$)—a composite measure involving activities such as getting into and out of a car, walking, and stair climbing (Podsiadlo & Richardson, 1991). Past evidence also indicates that performance on the up-and-go test can discriminate among various functional categories in older adults and is responsive to changes resulting from an increased level of physical activity (Podsiadlo & Richardson, 1991; Tinetti et al., 1986).

Studies conducted specifically on the 8-foot version of the up-and-go test indicate that it is an excellent discriminator of performance changes across age groups and that it can detect expected differences between high-active and low-active older adults. As seen in table 3.2, there was a consistent slowing of average times on the 8-foot up-and-go test for people in their 60s (5.2 seconds) compared to those in their 70s (6.1 seconds) and 80s (7.1 seconds). Table 3.3 shows that the average 8-foot up-and-go test scores of high-active older people were considerable faster (6.0 seconds) than those of the low-active group (7.1 seconds). The replication study conducted by Miotto et al. (1999) also indicated that the 8-foot up-and-go test scores of physically active older people were faster (4.9 seconds) than those of sedentary people (5.7 seconds).

Height and Weight

This test item measures participants' body mass index (BMI) and is included in the SFT to assess body weight relative to body height, a measure that is important because of its general relationship to body composition (especially the ratio of fat to lean muscle tissue). Generally, people with excess body fat relative to their muscle tissue will not be able to function (manage their bodies) as well as people with normal ratios of fat and muscle. Technically, BMI is determined by dividing weight in kilograms by height in meters squared (BMI = kg/m^2). An alternative formula, using nonmetric units, involves multiplying weight in pounds by 703 and dividing by height in inches squared: BMI = $(lbs \times 703)/in^2$. BMI can also be estimated using a conversion chart such as the one included in appendix F.

Although body mass index (BMI) is not a measure that was developed or validated for the SFT, we suggest that it be included as an indicator of functional fitness because of previous evidence showing its role in maintaining functional mobility. Studies show that individuals with high BMIs (or in some cases very low BMIs) are more likely to be disabled in later years than are people with normal body mass ratings (Galanos et al., 1994; Harris et al., 1989; Losonczy et al., 1995). High BMI values are also associated with numerous health problems including hypertension, heart disease, and Type II diabetes (U.S. Department of Health and Human Services, 1996), all of which also can have adverse effects on functional mobility.

Although experts have not determined the ideal BMI for older adults, partially due to the unknown changes that occur in muscle and bone during aging, the following are suggested as general guidelines (American College of Sports Medicine, 1998b; Evans & Rosenberg, 1991; Galanos et al., 1994; Harris et al., 1989; Losonczy et al., 1995; Shephard, 1997):

BMI = 19–26	Healthy range
≥ 27	Overweight, associated with increased risk for disease and loss of mobility
≤ 18	Underweight, could indicate loss of muscle mass and bone tissue

In summary, based on the related research, the results of studies conducted as part of the SFT project, the feedback from our expert review panels, and the recent findings in the Miotto et al. (1999) replication study, we believe that there is reasonably strong evidence in support of the SFT test items as valid measures of functional capacity in older adults. As indicated in chapter 2, it was our goal to provide documentation supporting at least two of the three major types of validity (content, criterion-referenced, or construct) for each test item, and we believe we have accomplished that goal. In addition to having acceptable validity, it also is important that test items have acceptable test-retest reliability. Procedures for estimating the test-retest reliability of the SFT items are presented in the following section.

RELIABILITY

Reliability, like validity, is an essential characteristic of a good test. A reliable test is one that produces scores that are relatively free of measurement error and are dependable and consistent from one trial to the next, even one day to the next, assuming that there are no changes in ability level or testing conditions (American Psychological Association, 1985). Obtaining stable (reliable) measures is critical whether tests are to be used by practitioners, for individual assessment, or for conducting research. A recommended method of estimating the reliability of a physical performance test is to give the test on two different days, usually two to five days apart, and then determine the correlation between the two sets of scores. A high correlation (greater than .80) between scores on day 1 and scores on day 2 indicates that the test has acceptable reliability, meaning that it produces scores that are relatively consistent from one time to the next (Safrit & Wood, 1995).

Procedures for Estimating Reliability

Because the reliability of a test can vary considerably depending on how and where a test is used, it is important that reliability studies be conducted for the specific population of interest and under conditions that are similar to those where the test is most likely to be given. Therefore, rather than depending on past research to support the reliability of the SFT, we conducted our own test-retest reliability studies using group testing conditions and trained volunteer assistants. Recall that the intent of the test is that it be easy to use in the field setting with minimal training of testing technicians.

Participants for the reliability study (82 men and women, mean age = 71.8 years) were solicited from a nearby retirement housing complex and from enrollees in the senior exercise classes at our university. All participants were independent-living, did not require a cane or other assistive device to walk, and had no medical conditions that would prohibit their participation in the testing. All tests were conducted by trained senior volunteers or by graduate student volunteers. Prior to all testing, participants performed 8 minutes of warm-up and stretching exercises. All tests and retests were administered two to five days apart. Because our pilot testing indicated that a practice trial was necessary in order to obtain stable scores on both the 6-minute walk test and the 2-minute step test, these items were administered on three different occasions, with the first test treated as a practice trial. The practice trial helps the participants establish an efficient pace for these tests, thus improving their scoring consistency on subsequent trials.

Reliability of the SFT Items

The test-retest reliability value for each test item was established by calculating the intraclass correlation coefficient (R) using a one-way analysis of variance (ANOVA) appropriate for establishing the reliability of a single trial (Baumgartner & Jackson, 1999). The one-way ANOVA model treats all sources of measurement variation, including changes in day-to-day performance, as error (lack of reliability), thus resulting in the most accurate estimate of stability reliability. Results indicate that the test-retest correlation values for the SFT items ranged from .80 to .98, indicating acceptable reliability for all test items (Rikli & Jones, 1999a). See table 3.4 for specific R values and 95% confidence intervals for each test item. According to APA standards (American Psychological Association, 1985), confidence intervals should always be reported along with R values as an aid in their interpretation. In reality, any single R value is just the best estimate of the true R value, with the true value expected to fall within the given confidence interval.

Table 3.4 Test-Retest Reliability (*r*) and 95% Confidence Intervals (CI) for Senior Fitness Test Items

Test item	All participants			Men			Women		
	r	(CI)	*n*	*r*	(CI)	*n*	*r*	(CI)	*n*
Chair stand	.89	(.79–.93)	76	.86	(.77–.90)	34	.92	(.87–.95)	42
Arm curl	.81	(.72–.88)	78	.81	(.66–.90)	36	.80	(.67–.89)	42
6-min walk	.94	(.90–.96)	66	.97	(.92–.99)	23	.91	(.84–.95)	43
2-min step	.90	(.84–.93)	78	.90	(.80–.95)	36	.89	(.83–.94)	42
Chair sit-and-reach	.95	(.92–.97)	76	.92	(.85–.96)	34	.96	(.93–.98)	42
Back scratch	.96	(.94–.98)	77	.96	(.93–.98)	35	.92	(.86–.96)	42
8-ft up-and-go	.95	(.92–.97)	76	.98	(.96–.99)	34	.90	(.83–.95)	42

Reprinted from Rikli and Jones 1999.

In addition to being valid and reliable, it also is important that tests have some type of performance standards that can be used in evaluating test results. The next section describes the procedures followed in developing these standards for the SFT.

PERFORMANCE STANDARDS

Performance standards can be either norm-referenced or criterion-referenced. Standards that provide a basis for comparing an individual's scores to others within a particular group are referred to as norm-referenced standards or norms. Test norms are statistics that summarize the typical performance of a specific population of individuals. Criterion-referenced standards, on the other hand, identify scores that are associated with or "referenced to" a particular category of health or performance. In developing the SFT, our goal was to establish normative standards and to begin to identify the threshold (criterion) scores on the test items that are associated with being at risk for loss of functional mobility.

Establishing Norm-Referenced Standards

Normative scores are developed by testing a large number of people in a specifically defined population, then summarizing the data using descriptive statistics. A common method of organizing normative data is through the use of percentile tables. Percentile tables indicate the percentile equivalent (rank) associated with any given raw score. Raw scores are those scores received directly from each test item, such as the number of yards covered during the 6-minute walk test or the number of repetitions completed in 30 seconds on the arm curl test. A raw score falling at the midpoint of a distribution for a specific age group would be equivalent to the 50th percentile in that distribution, meaning that 50% of those tested scored below that particular score and 50% scored above it. Similarly, a raw score falling at the 75th percentile would indicate that 75% of the population scored below that value, with only 25% scoring above it. In the SFT, percentile scores are reported separately for men and women in five-year age groups from 60 to 94. The following section describes the procedures and results of the nationwide study that was conducted to establish normative scores for the SFT (Rikli & Jones, 1999b).

Normative Study Procedures

Testing for the normative study took place over an 18-month period during 1997 and 1998. Test sites for collecting the data were solicited through announcements made at various professional meetings and workshops and through notices placed in magazines, newspapers, and journals. The older adult participants at each site were solicited through a call for volunteers made at various senior centers and similar community locations and through local newspapers, radio, and television.

To be included in the study, participants had to be community-residing, independent-living, ambulatory without regular use of assistive devices, and have no medical conditions that prohibited them from participating in the tests. The official study sample included 7,183 volunteer participants (5,048 women and 2,135 men), ages 60 to 94, from 267 test sites in 21 different states. A summary of participant characteristics is presented in table 3.5.

To maximize consistency of the testing procedures, a large emphasis was placed on training test administrators and assistants. Training workshops were held for most of the lead coordinators from each of the participating states. State coordinators, in turn, held training workshops for local technicians and assistants. A testing manual and an instructional videotape, given to all testing personnel, provided an additional source of information and training.

Testing typically took place in a group setting with up to 24 participants per group. The tests were administered circuit-style in six stations that were set up around the periphery of a large multipurpose room. Following an 8- to 10-minute warm-up, participants were divided evenly among the six stations to begin the tests. To minimize the effects of fatigue, stations were arranged in the following order: (1) chair stand test, (2) arm curl test, (3) height and weight and 2-minute step test, (4) chair sit-and-reach test, (5) back scratch test, and (6) 8-foot up-and-go test. A diagram of the circuit setup for group testing can be found in chapter 4, figure 4.11. As indicated, when the 2-minute step test was used to assess aerobic endurance instead of the 6-minute walk test (usually due to lack of space or to inclement weather), it was included as part of the height and weight station. If, the 6-minute walk test was used as the test of aerobic endurance, it was administered as a group after all other tests had been completed. A detailed description of testing procedures can be found in an article by Rikli and Jones (1999b).

Study Results/Participant Characteristics

Data from the study provided percentile-based normative performance scores for men and women separately in five-year age groups from 60 to 94. The percentile score equivalents for raw scores on all test items are presented in the normative percentile tables in appendix H. A percentile rank represents that point in a distribution of scores below which that given percent of scores fall. A raw score falling at the 25th percentile, for example, indicates that 25% of the scores in that particular age group would be lower than that score while 75% would be higher. Chapter 5 contains tables of the normal range of scores for men and women (see tables 5.3 and 5.4), which provides an alternative, more user-friendly way of looking at the normative data. These tables present only the normal ranges of scores, defined as those representing the middle 50% for each age and gender group on each test

Table 3.5 Participant Characteristics: Means and Standard Deviations (in parentheses)

	Age groups							
	Combined	60–64	65–69	70–74	75–79	80–84	85–89	90–94
Total # of subjects	7,183	861	1,566	1,813	1,451	784	470	234
Women	5,048	620	1,084	1,298	987	543	354	158
Men	2,135	241	482	515	464	241	116	76
Mean age (years)								
Women	73.3	62.1	67.1	72.0	76.8	81.4	86.1	92.0
	(7.6)	(1.5)	(1.4)	(1.4)	(1.4)	(1.2)	(1.1)	(2.1)
Men	73.4	62.2	67.1	72.1	76.9	81.4	86.0	92.3
	(7.4)	(1.4)	(1.4)	(1.5)	(1.4)	(1.1)	(1.0)	(1.9)
Height (inches)								
Women	63.2	64.0	63.7	63.4	62.9	62.4	62.2	61.1
	(2.8)	(2.7)	(2.8)	(2.7)	(2.7)	(2.7)	(2.6)	(3.1)
Men	68.7	69.4	69.3	68.8	68.5	68.1	67.6	66.5
	(3.1)	(2.9)	(3.2)	(3.1)	(2.9)	(3.1)	(3.0)	(3.3)
Weight (pounds)								
Women	146.5	153.6	153.3	149.7	142.9	136.8	134.0	128.2
	(28.4)	(32.4)	(30.5)	(27.4)	(24.6)	(23.1)	(22.0)	(23.7)
Men	178.8	187.6	187.5	178.8	176.4	172.6	161.9	155.5
	(28.5)	(31.0)	(30.1)	(26.5)	(26.6)	(24.9)	(22.9)	(20.5)
Education (# of years)	14.5	14.8	14.5	14.4	14.5	14.4	14.6	14.9
	(3.3)	(2.9)	(2.9)	(3.0)	(2.9)	(2.9)	(3.2)	(3.9)
Chronic conditions (#)	1.7	1.4	1.5	1.6	1.9	2.0	2.0	2.1
	(1.4)	(1.3)	(1.3)	(1.3)	(1.4)	(1.4)	(1.4)	(1.8)
Medications (# of prescriptions)	1.6	1.1	1.4	1.5	1.7	1.8	1.9	1.7
	(1.6)	(1.4)	(1.6)	(1.6)	(1.6)	(1.6)	(1.6)	(1.7)
Quality of life (1 = very low; 7 = very high)	5.3	5.5	5.4	5.3	5.3	5.1	5.1	5.1
	(1.0)	(1.0)	(1.0)	(.9)	(.9)	(1.0)	(1.0)	(1.1)
Depression (1 = none; 7 = severe)	2.0	2.1	2.0	2.0	2.1	2.1	2.1	1.9
	(1.0)	(1.0)	(0.9)	(1.0)	(1.0)	(1.1)	(1.2)	(0.9)
Moderate exercise (%) (≥3 days/week)	65.3	69.2	70.1	69.2	63.8	58.7	54.0	46.0
Self-reported health								
Very good	56.9	65.0	64.7	57.7	53.6	47.2	44.7	49.5
Good	34.1	27.7	28.4	34.8	36.6	40.8	42.3	34.7
Fair	9.0	7.3	6.9	7.5	9.8	12.0	13.0	16.4
Functional level (%)*								
Advanced	47.4	66.6	58.8	51.9	42.2	30.1	21.0	14.0
Moderate	35.4	25.4	32.7	35.0	42.0	40.0	40.1	28.5
Low	17.2	8.0	8.5	13.1	15.8	29.9	38.9	57.5

(continued)

Table 3.5 *(continued)*

	Age groups							
	Combined	60–64	65–69	70–74	75–79	80–84	85–89	90–94
Ethnicity (%)								
Caucasian	89.1	80.0	87.5	88.2	92.6	94.2	94.5	90.2
African American	2.5	4.7	2.3	2.1	2.0	1.6	3.0	2.8
Hispanic	4.2	8.0	5.4	5.4	2.6	.9	.8	2.1
Other	4.2	7.3	4.8	4.3	2.7	3.3	1.6	4.9

* Functional ratings were based on responses to a 12-item Composite Physical Function scale (Rikli & Jones, 1998) asking participants to indicate their ability to perform common everyday activities ranging from personal care items such as bathing and dressing oneself (basic activities of daily living—ADLs), to various household, gardening, walking, and lifting activities (activities needed to live independently within the community—IADLs), to advanced activities such as moving heavy objects, sports, and aerobic dance activities (strenuous exercise). Advanced functioning participants were those who could perform all 12 items with no difficulty. Moderate functioning were defined as those that could perform 7 of the 12 items with no difficulty. Low-functioning individuals could perform six or fewer of the tasks with no difficulty or assistance. Specifically, low-functioning individuals could *not* perform without difficulty at least three common IADLs, such as walking half a mile, lifting and carrying 10 pounds (equivalent to a full bag of groceries), and household activities such as scrubbing floors and vacuuming.

Reprinted from Rikli and Jones 1999.

item, that is, scores that fall between the 25th and 75th percentiles. Scores higher than the normal range are interpreted as above normal, while lower scores are interpreted as below normal.

Data from the SFT normative study also provide important information on the typical amounts and rates of declines experienced by this cross section of older adults. As illustrated in figure 3.1, the data reveal remarkably consistent patterns of declines in physical performance scores over most five-year age groups for both men and women on all test items. Statistical analysis of these data indicate that the average decline across the majority of the adjacent five-year age groups was statistically significant for both men and women (Rikli & Jones, 1999b). The overall amount of decline across variables from age 60 to age 94 was in the 30% to 45% range, resulting in an approximate 1% to 1.5% per year or 10% to 15% per decade loss in strength, endurance, and agility/balance. The exact percent of decline was not calculated for the two flexibility tests since the measurement scales involved an arbitrarily determined zero point, thus making it inappropriate to conduct ratio types of calculations. Exact means and standard deviations for all variables can be found in Rikli and Jones, 1999b.

As also can be observed in figure 3.1, the pattern and amount of decline across ages is similar for men and women. However, there are definite gender differences on the test items, with men consistently scoring better than women on the strength, endurance, and agility/balance tests and women consistently performing better than men on the two flexibility measures. These gender differences were significant across all age groups on all test items (Rikli and Jones, 1999b).

Again, it is important to remember that these normative scores represent average amounts of decline within each age group and can be quite different for different subgroups of people. As shown in figure 3.2, for example, older adults who regularly participate in physical activity have overall better scoring distributions than those who are less active, with almost all comparisons being highly significant (Jones & Rikli, 1999). Further, not only were the scores of active people higher to begin with, but the average rate of decline in performance between age

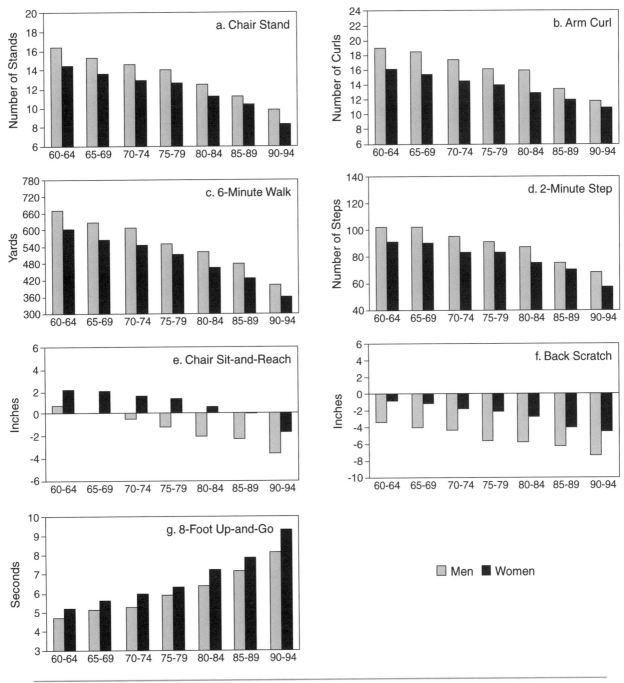

Figure 3.1 Fitness mean scores across five-year age groups for men and women.
Reprinted from Rikli & Jones 1999.

60 to 94 was smaller for the active than for the inactive participants (31% versus 44%).

The data suggest that for sedentary individuals, approximately 50% of the decline in performance might have been offset by being active. To illustrate, look at the chair stand test data in figure 3.2a. Over the three decades from the early 60s to the early 90s, the chair stand test performance of inactive individuals declines by about 7 points, from an average score of approximately 14 to an average score of approximately 7. However, by age 90, scores of active individuals are 3.5 points

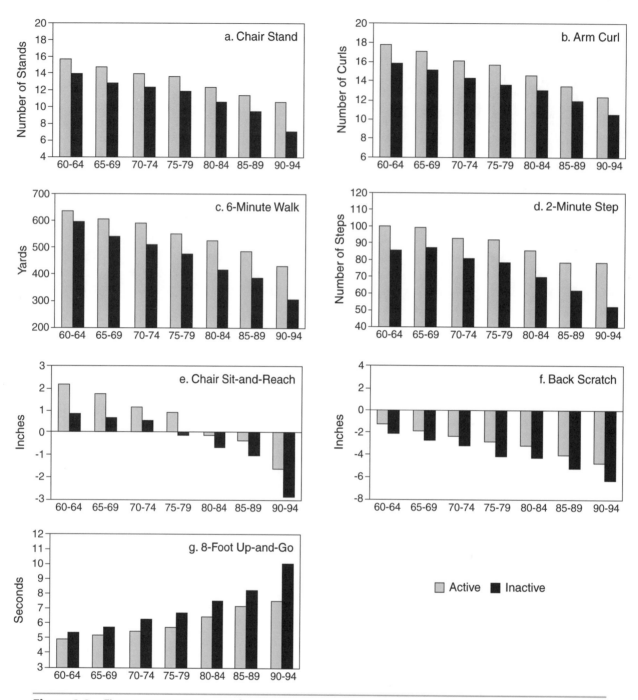

Figure 3.2 Fitness test scores across five-year age groups for active and inactive participants.

higher (the exact mean is 10.5 as reported in Rikli & Jones, 1999a), thus indicating that 50% of the loss in lower-body strength experienced by inactive individuals might have been alleviated had they been active. In other words, instead of declining from a score of 14 to a score of 7, by becoming active, the formerly inactive person might have declined only to a score of 10.5 (a 3.5-point loss instead of a 7-point loss in chair stand test performance).

In calculating similar "savings ratios" for the other fitness items, we find that the average percent of loss that might have been saved by being active is 52%.

This statistic is especially important when considering that a 50% reduction in age-related decline translates, over a 30-year period, into a 15-year "fitness advantage" for active compared to inactive people. Such statistics are in line with several other studies in suggesting that regular participation in moderate physical activity can reduce physical decline by 50% and delay age-related physical deterioration by 10 to 20 years (Chandler & Hadley, 1996; Lacroix et al., 1993; Morey et al., 1998; Seeman et al., 1995; Shephard, 1997; Stewart et al., 1994). Or, put another way, our data and others suggest that sedentary people tend to experience twice as much physical loss as active people.

Of special concern in interpreting data and especially in using normative standards to interpret individual scores are the characteristics of the study (normative) population. As indicated in table 3.5, the participants in this study were 89.1% Caucasian, 4.2% Hispanic, 2.5% African American, and 4.2% from other groups (2.3% of which were Asian). These proportions are fairly close to U.S. national statistics except for the African American population, which is underrepresented in our study, and the "other" population, which is slightly overrepresented. The actual racial/ethnic percentages in the United States for the 65+ population are 86.7% Caucasian, 3.7% Hispanic, 8.0% African American, and 1.6% "other" (U.S. Bureau of the Census, 1996).

Overall, the participants in the study were independent-living well educated (all age groups reporting averaging more than 14 years of education), were generally active (over 50% in most age categories reported that they participated at least three times per week for at least 30 minutes a day in moderate activity), were generally healthy, considered their life to be of high quality, had low levels of depression, and generally reported moderate to high levels of functional ability well into their 70s and early 80s. Although the characteristics of the volunteer participants in the SFT study surely are different from the entire population of older adults, they do not differ greatly from the data reported in other similar large-scale samples of independent-living, community-residing older adults, such as in the Baltimore Longitudinal Study of Aging—LSOA (Rakowski & Mor, 1992), the Established Populations for Epidemiologic Studies of the Elderly—EPESE (Schoenfeld, Malmrose, Blazer, Gold, & Seeman, 1994; Seeman et al., 1994; Simonsick, et al., 1993), and the National Health and Nutrition Examination Survey—NHANES (Hubert, Bloch, & Fries, 1993).

In the SFT study, for example, the self-reported rate of participation in moderate-level physical activity was 65% compared to 68% reported in the EPESE population (Simonsick et al., 1993), and 58% in the NHANES data (Hubert et al., 1993). Relative to health status, 91% of the SFT participants reported their health as good, very good, or excellent compared to 70% in the LSOA data (Rakowski & Mor, 1992) and 73.2% in the EPESE studies (Schoenfeld et al., 1994). However, the participants in the LSOA and EPESE studies were all over 70 years of age rather than over 60, as in our study. The number of chronic health conditions (average = 1.3) reported in the NHANES data for participants with a mean age of 62.2 (Hubert et al., 1993) is nearly identical to the 1.4 average number of health conditions reported by the 60- to 64-year-olds in the SFT study. Also, the average of 1.7 health conditions reported across all age groups in the SFT study appears to be fairly consistent to EPESE statistics indicating that 63% had fewer than two health conditions, with only 37% having two or more (Schoenfeld et al., 1994; Seeman et al., 1994).

One area in which participants in the SFT study may differ significantly from those in other studies is level of education. SFT participants reported an average of 14.5 years of education, which would be equivalent to 2.5 years of post high school education. Statistics on both the LSOA and EPESE subjects indicate that only 47% had 12 or more years of education (Rakowski & Mor, 1992; Schoenfeld et al., 1994).

Overall, participants in the SFT study do not appear to vary greatly from those in other large-scale community-based studies, suggesting that the normative results of this study should be generalizable to other similar groups of older adults. However, care must be taken when using SFT norms for interpreting scores of individuals that are different from those represented in these studies. It is important to remember that the SFT was designed for independent-living, community-residing older adults and that the test norms are based on a volunteer sample from this population. Using volunteers in studies results in a sample of convenience, rather than a sample that is a true representation of the entire population of interest. Convenience samples almost always are healthier and higher functioning than the population as a whole. However, since the SFT participant characteristics are fairly similar to other volunteer groups of older adults, the norms should provide reasonable standards of comparison for the majority of people most likely to take the test— willing participants in various community programs, individual testing programs, or research studies.

In addition to establishing norm-referenced standards, data from the SFT study also provided a basis for beginning to establish criterion-referenced standards for the various test items. In developing the SFT, we especially were interested in identifying possible threshold values that would signify being at risk for losing functional mobility.

Establishing Criterion-Referenced Standards

Criterion-referenced standards are developed by identifying scores that are associated with a particular goal or category of interest, such as being healthy or being functionally independent. In many cases, criterion-referenced standards provide more important types of information than do norm-referenced standards. For a 60-year-old man, for example, knowing that his cholesterol level is average for his age group is much less important than knowing whether it does or does not place him at risk for cardiac problems.

Relative to the SFT, we believe that important information can be gained from both norm-referenced and criterion-referenced standards. Normative standards provide a basis for evaluating one's fitness level, particularly one's rate of change in fitness level over the years, relative to other people of the same age. Criterion standards, on the other hand, can be helpful in identifying the fitness level needed to maintain functional independence. Because setting criterion-referenced standards involves referencing a particular score to a particular criterion condition, such as functional ability, it is important to understand how the criterion condition is defined and evaluated.

Defining Functional Ability

Because a goal in developing the SFT was to identify the threshold fitness scores associated with being at risk for losing one's ability to function independently, it was important that, in addition to testing participants' fitness levels, we also assessed their functional ability levels. Specifically, functional ability was assessed through self-evaluation using a composite physical functional (CPF) scale that had previously been evaluated for reliability and validity (Rikli & Jones, 1998). The 12-item CPF was designed to assess function across a wide range of abilities—from basic activities of daily living (ADLs; e.g., dressing and bathing oneself) to intermediate or instrumental activities of daily living (IADLs; e.g., housework and shopping) to advanced activities such as strenuous household, sport, and exercise activities.

CPF scores were used to categorize individuals as either high functioning or low functioning, with high functioning being those who indicated that they could perform all 12 items with no difficulty and low functioning being those who could perform no more than 50% (6 or fewer) of the tasks without difficulty. More specifically, low-functioning individuals were those who were unable to perform without difficulty at least three or more common IADL activities associated with the ability to live independently within the community—lifting 10 pounds, walking half a mile, climbing a flight of stairs, and doing routine household activities such as vacuuming and scrubbing floors. As seen in table 3.5, there were both low- and high-functioning people within each age group from 60-64 to 90-94. The clear trend, of course, was for a gradual decrease over the years in the percent of people who evaluated themselves as high functioning and a gradual increase in the percent who considered themselves low functioning. Of special interest to this discussion, however, is the fitness level that is associated with being low functioning and potentially at risk for loss of physical independence.

Identifying Criterion Reference Points Associated With Loss of Functional Mobility

The data in the SFT study revealed a strong positive association between fitness level and self-reported functional ability level, with higher-fit scores being associated with high functional ability and low-fit scores associated with low functional ability (Rikli & Jones, 2000). Although far from being conclusive, the average fitness scores of those who reported having difficulties with common everyday activities associated with independent living (e.g., lifting 10 pounds, walking half a mile, climbing stairs, or doing housework) provide a type of threshold value or criterion reference point that is associated with loss of functional mobility. Table 3.6 presents the average fitness scores associated with high and low levels

Table 3.6 Fitness Means and Standard Deviations (in parentheses) for Men and Women With High and Low Levels of Functional Ability

Test item	Self-reported functional ability			
	High ability		Low ability	
	Men	Women	Men	Women
Chair stand (# of stands)	15.5 (4.2)	14.1 (3.6)	8.3 (3.4)	8.4 (4.1)
Arm curl (# of reps)	18.0 (4.9)	15.7 (4.6)	10.8 (3.5)	11.0 (3.9)
6-min walk (yd)	636 (96)	589 (84)	360 (138)	362 (135)
2-min step (# of steps)	100 (24)	94 (24)	65 (25)	65 (25)
Chair sit-and-reach (in.)	0.2 (4.5)	2.4 (3.6)	−3.8 (4.8)	−1.9 (4.1)
Back scratch (in.)	−4.0 (4.7)	−0.9 (3.5)	−8.0 (5.7)	−4.5 (4.7)
8-ft up-and-go (sec)	5.1 (1.2)	5.5 (1.1)	8.9 (2.9)	8.8 (3.2)

of self-reported functional ability. Also, performance charts indicating the at-risk scoring zones associated with loss of function are presented in chapter 5. The ability to identify and hopefully rehabilitate low levels of physical performance is particularly important in light of several recent studies showing that, in fact, low fitness is a prime predictor of subsequent disability in later years (Gill et al., 1996; Gill, Williams, & Tinetti, 1995; Guralnik et al., 1995; Morey et al., 1998).

Admittedly, these initial criterion values are rather loosely defined and need further research to confirm their validity. In the meantime, however, we believe these figures can provide useful, and previously unavailable, guidelines (reference points) for interpreting physical ability in older adults. Test users also are cautioned that the threshold scores used to describe the at-risk zones were developed based on group averages and may not apply to all individuals. Individuals who are very small, for example, may not score well compared to others of their age group but may, in fact, be quite capable of managing their own bodies and their own environments.

SUMMARY

Published tests should be valid and reliable and should have accompanying performance standards to aid in the interpretation of test scores. Ideally, tests should be validated using multiple sources of evidence including content-related, criterion-related, and construct-related evidence.

In developing the SFT, content (logical) evidence regarding the relevance of the selected fitness categories was provided through literature review and through expert opinion, most of which was reported in chapter 2 in the discussions on Conceptual Background and Functional Fitness Parameters. Criterion-related evidence was documented by showing the correlation (r values) between performance on each test item and performance on a recognized criterion measure, when an appropriate criterion could be identified. As indicated in table 3.1, the correlation values ranged from .71 to .84, indicating moderately good criterion validity. Construct-related validity, determined through the "group differences" method (Safrit & Wood, 1995), was evidenced by the test item's ability to detect expected performance differences from one age group to another (table 3.2) and between people with high versus low levels of physical activity (table 3.3).

The test-retest reliability of the SFT was assessed using intraclass correlation (R) procedures to compare test scores on day 1 with retest scores on day 2. Studies to assess SFT reliability were designed specifically to reflect conditions similar to those where most testing is likely to take place, that is, in a group setting within the community, using trained volunteer assistants. As shown in table 3.4, test-retest R values for the test items range from .80 and .97, indicating acceptable reliability for all items.

Performance standards for the SFT are based on a nationwide study involving over 7,000 older adults from 267 testing sites in 21 states. Data from the study provide age group normative standards (reported in percentiles) for men and women ages 60 to 94. Test users are reminded that the SFT norms are based on a volunteer sample of independent-living older adults who are healthier, better educated, and more active than the total population of older adults. The characteristics of the SFT participants are, however, similar to other large-scale samples of community-residing older adults and therefore appear to provide relevant standards of comparison for the majority of people most likely to take the test—that is, willing participants residing within the community.

Test users are further reminded that the norms represent average scores of broad ranges of ability levels and that the performance of subgroups of older adults might be expected to vary considerably. The men and women in the study who participated in regular physical activity, for example, had considerably higher scores on all test items in every age group than did people who were inactive or less active.

Finally, the data also provided a basis for beginning to develop criterion-referenced standards for the SFT. Specifically, the average fitness scores of participants reporting low levels of functional ability (i.e., those having difficulty with normal everyday activities) provide a type of threshold value or criterion reference point associated with loss of functional mobility. Although further research is needed to validate these reference points, we believe that the data provide some important, previously unavailable guidelines for interpreting physical ability level in older adults. Chapter 5 contains additional information on using the SFT performance tables and charts to interpret individual test scores.

In the next chapter we will describe the procedures for administering and scoring the SFT items. Included will be information needed to properly prepare participants for testing, checklists for gathering supplies and equipment, descriptions of the specific testing and scoring protocols, and guidelines for conducting group testing and for training volunteer assistants.

4

TEST ADMINISTRATION

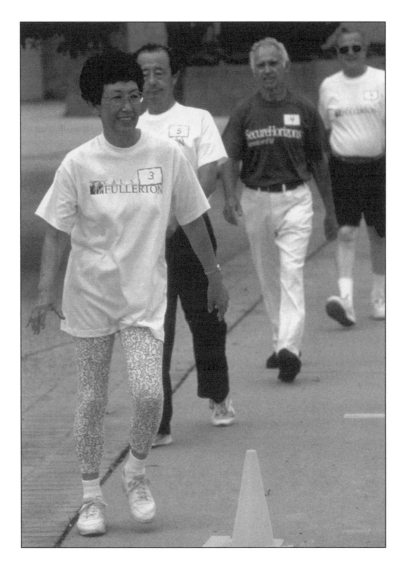

Establishing Consistent Testing Protocols

The Senior Fitness Test (SFT) was designed to be easy to administer in common community settings without extensive time, equipment, technical expertise, or space requirements. The complete test battery can be given in approximately 30 minutes to an individual or to pairs of individuals, using partners to assist with scoring. However, we also designed the test to be easily administered to a group of participants (up to 24 at a time) within a 60- to 90-minute period with the help of trained assistants.

In previous chapters we described the rationale for the SFT, possible uses of the SFT, and why each physical parameter is important for keeping people active and independent in later years. In this chapter we will provide you with detailed instructions for planning and administering the test items and will discuss guidelines for group testing. More specifically, the topics will include the following:

- Pretest procedures and considerations
- Administering the tests
- Guidelines for group testing

PRETEST PROCEDURES AND CONSIDERATIONS

Although the SFT is comparatively simple to administer and score, as with any test, careful planning will be required to ensure reliable testing protocols and meaningful data. The following is a list of pretesting procedures and conditions that need to be addressed before the test day. Attention to these points is important to assure participant safety, testing efficiency, and accurate measurements.

1. Technician training. Those administering the test items should be properly trained and well practiced regarding the testing procedures—that is, they should understand and be able to follow the exact protocols for administering the tests and recording the scores. Strict adherence to the established test procedures is essential if meaningful comparisons are to be made to the normative standards, or if comparisons are to be made from one testing time to another, such as before and after initiating an exercise program. After becoming familiar with the test instructions contained in this chapter, technicians should engage in ample practice testing prior to actually giving the tests to clients.

2. Informed consent/assumption of liability. If test results are being used for research purposes, the examiner must obtain informed consent from the participants prior to testing. The purpose of obtaining informed consent is to protect the rights of human subjects, that is, to assure that they have been informed of the test's purposes and risks and are aware of their right to discontinue testing at any time. Although a signed informed consent form may not be required in your program, we recommend that it (or something similar) be used anyway as a way of explaining the risks and responsibilities associated with testing. A sample informed consent/assumption of liability form describing testing purposes, risks, protocols, and individual rights and responsibilities is included in appendix A.

3. Screening of participants. Although the test items are safe to administer to most community-residing older adults without medical screening, there are some exceptions. People who should *not* participate in testing without physician approval are those who

- have been advised by their doctors not to exercise because of a medical condition;

- have had congestive heart failure;
- are currently experiencing joint pain, chest pain, dizziness, or have exertional angina (chest tightness, pressure, pain, heaviness) during exercise; or
- have uncontrolled high blood pressure (greater than 160/100).

As part of the information you normally obtain from your clients (name, address, emergency contact, health background, etc.), you should also explain the previously listed conditions and ask clients to obtain medical clearance from their doctor if needed. Asking clients to sign an informed consent/assumption of liability form that describes these conditions (see appendix A) is one way of communicating this information. A sample medical clearance form, should it be required, is included in appendix B.

4. Pretest instructions to participants. To ensure maximum safety and performance, participants also should be given information prior to test day concerning the best way to prepare for testing. Specifically, participants should be asked to

- avoid strenuous physical activity one or two days prior to assessment;
- avoid excess alcohol use for 24 hours prior to testing;
- eat a light meal one hour prior to testing;
- wear clothing and shoes appropriate for participating in physical activity;
- bring a hat and sunglasses for walking outside, and reading glasses (if needed) for completing forms;
- bring the informed consent and medical clearance forms, if required; and
- inform the test administrator of any medical conditions or medications that could affect performance.

Also, to improve their scoring accuracy, participants need to practice taking the aerobic endurance test prior to the test day. They should time themselves either walking for six minutes or stepping for two minutes. Practicing the test will help them determine the pace that will work best for them. The informed consent and medical clearance forms, if needed, should be distributed to clients at the same time as the list of participant instructions. A copy-ready example of a participant instructions form is included in appendix C. You may copy or adapt this form, as needed, for use in your program.

5. Testing equipment/supplies. All testing equipment and supplies should be gathered and readily available prior to testing. Most of the materials required for the SFT are common items that can be found in most exercise facilities, can be brought from home, or can be obtained easily at local stores. Table 4.1 contains a list of all equipment and supplies needed to conduct the SFT, along with possible vendors/sources where they can be obtained. Specific uses of each equipment/supply item is indicated in the test item descriptions in the next section.

6. Data recording forms (scorecards). Forms for recording the test scores, similar to the sample shown in figure 4.1, should be prepared prior to testing. The "comments" line on the scorecard is for indicating any deviations from proper protocol. Scores obtained from adjusted protocols, of course, should not be compared to the normative standards but can be used for individual comparisons from one testing time to the next. A copy-ready form of the scorecard is included in appendix D. Note that the information appears twice on the same page, thus allowing it to be copied onto heavy paper and then cut in half to form two approximately 5" × 8" scoring cards.

Table 4.1   Vendors/Sources for SFT Equipment and Supplies

Equipment/supply items*	Possible vendor/source
Folding chairs Stopwatches Hand weights (5- & 8-lb dumbbells) Scale Masking tape 30" cord Long tape measure (≥20 yards) 4 cones (or similar markers)	Generally available at major discount stores such as K-Mart, Target, & Wal-Mart. Can also check Sears & local sports stores.
Popsicle sticks (for counting laps on 6-min walk) 60" tape measure 18" ruler (half a yardstick)	Usually available in craft/fabric sections of above discount stores or in specialty craft/fabric stores.
Tally counter† (for 2-min step test) Small pencils Name tags 3" × 5" cards (may be used as alternate way of marking laps in 6-min walk)	Available in discount office supply stores such as Office Depot, Staples, & OfficeMax
Individual score cards (approx. 5" × 8")	Information in appendix D can be copied onto 8 1/2 × 11 card stock, then cut in half.
Station signs (for use in group testing)	Information in appendix G can be copied onto heavy paper. Could also be mounted and laminated (at Kinkos) if so desired.

* For group testing, multiple numbers of some items will be required. See table 4.2.

† Purchase information for tally counters at time of publication is as follows:
   Office Depot: Available in stores only @ $8.99 (SKU #165-768)
   OfficeMax: Available as special order only @ $7.99; Call 1-800-788-8080 (SPR #24100)
   Staples: Available through phone order @ $9.99; Call 1-800-333-3330 (Item #BAT-9841000) or in stores @ $9.49 (SKU #211-821)

7. Testing order. In planning testing order it is important to consider whether you will be using the 6-minute walk test or the 2-minute step test as the aerobic endurance measure. If the 2-minute step test is used, the test items should be scheduled in the following order to minimize fatigue: chair stand test, arm curl test, 2-minute step test, chair sit-and-reach test, back scratch test, and 8-foot up-and-go test. If the 6-minute walk test is used, it should be administered last after all other tests have been completed. Normally, if the 6-minute test is given, the 2-minute step test is omitted from the above rotation. If you choose to give both the 2-minute step test and the 6-minute walk, we recommend that the 6-minute walk be administered on a separate day to avoid over fatiguing the participants. The height and weight measurements can be taken at any time, since they involve no exertion of effort. During group testing we recommend that the height and weight measures be scheduled at station number three, along with the 2-minute step test if it is given or instead of the 2-minute step test if it is omitted.

8. Environmental conditions. The tests should not be administered if the temperature or humidity conditions are uncomfortable or appear unsafe for

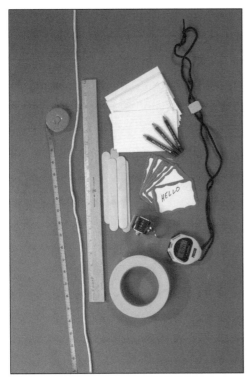 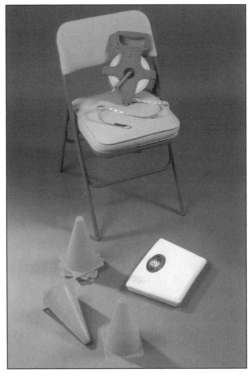

Equipment and supplies you will need to administer the SFT.

Scorecard: Senior Fitness Test

Date ___2/12/01___

Name ___Mary Jacob___   M___ F _√_ Age __76__ Ht _61"_ Wt _129_

Test Item	Trial 1	Trial 2	Comments
1. Chair Stand Test (# in 30 sec)	15	N/A	
2. Arm Curl Test (# in 30 sec)	10	N/A	*Had difficulty keeping good form—needs work on upper-body strength*
3. 2-Minute Step Test* (# of steps)	520 yd	N/A	
4. Chair Sit-and-Reach Test (nearest 1/2 in.: +/-)	+1.5	+2.0	Extended leg: ®or L
5. Back Scratch Test (nearest 1/2 in.: +/-)	-4.5	-3.0	Hand over: ®or L shoulder
6. 8-Ft Up-and-Go Test (nearest 1/10 sec)	6.1	6.3	
6- Minute Walk Test (# of yd)	___	N/A	

* Omit 2-minute step test if 6-minute walk test is given.

Figure 4.1 Sample scorecard.

the participants. Because individuals differ substantially with respect to their temperature/humidity tolerance, the best guide is each person's own comfort level. Always watch for signs of overheating or overexertion and stop the test immediately if symptoms occur or if the participant requests to stop.

9. Signs of overexertion. The following are common physiological signs associated with overheating or overexertion. Testing should be stopped immediately if any of the following conditions appear:

- Unusual fatigue or shortness of breath
- Dizziness or lightheadedness
- Tightness or pain in chest
- Irregular heartbeats
- Pain of any kind
- Numbness
- Loss of muscle control or balance
- Nausea or vomiting
- Confusion or disorientation
- Blurred vision

10. Emergency procedures/accident reporting. Before you begin testing, be sure to plan procedures that will be followed in case of emergency. Know where the closest phone is and be sure that emergency procedures and phone numbers are posted clearly. It also is a good idea to have typed directions to your facility posted nearby in case you should need to call for emergency assistance. If any kind of injury or illness occurs during testing, you should complete an accident report describing the situation and the procedures that were followed. A sample accident report form is included in appendix E.

ADMINISTERING THE TESTS

This section describes the procedures that should be followed on test day. Included is information on proper warm-up and the pretest instructions that should be given to participants before they begin the tests. Also presented are detailed descriptions of each of the official SFT protocols.

Warm-Up Exercises and Participant Instructions

Before testing begins, participants should engage in five to eight minutes of warm-up and stretching activities. It doesn't really matter what specific activities are used during the warm-up, as long as they involve the large-muscle groups and are not too strenuous. Activities that involve marching in place, swinging the arms, and up-and-back and side-to-side walking steps are good ways to warm up the muscles. Performing these activities to music can make them more enjoyable and provide a fun way to begin the testing experience. After the warm-up, some simple stretches should be done, paying special attention to the areas that will be stretched during the tests, especially the lower-body (hamstring) muscles and the upper-body (shoulder) area. Sample exercises that stretch the major muscles and joints involved in the testing are illustrated in figure 4.2.

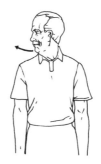

a) Head Turns. Slowly turn your head to the right until you feel gentle tension on the side of your neck, hold five seconds, then slowly turn your head to center and repeat the stretch to the left side.

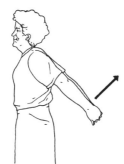

b) Head Half Circles. Slowly tilt your head over to the right side until you feel gentle tension, then slowly rotate your head forward and to the left side. Repeat the stretch on the opposite side.

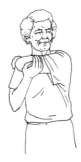

c) Single Arm Crossover. Using your left hand, grab your right arm and slowly pull it across your chest until you feel gentle tension, hold five seconds, and repeat with your left arm.

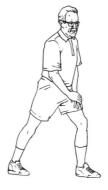

d) Chest Stretch. Grasp hands behind your back and slowly lift your arms up behind your back until you feel gentle tension in your chest, shoulders, and arms; hold five seconds.

e) Calf Stretch. Step forward with your left foot, keeping your feet parallel to each other. Shift your body weight forward by bending your left knee, keeping your right leg straight and your heel on the floor. Hold 10 seconds and repeat with your right foot forward.

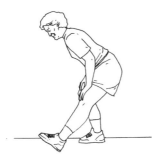

f) Hamstring Stretch. Extend your left leg forward with your foot lightly flexed, then bend your right knee and lean forward from the hips, using your hands for support. Keep leaning forward until you feel gentle tension in back of your left leg. Hold 10 seconds and repeat with your right leg forward. Be sure to keep your back straight, not rounded.

Figure 4.2 Examples of stretching exercises to use prior to administering the SFT.

Guidelines for Stretching

Do:

- Perform some type of warm-up activity prior to stretching (to increase circulation and body temperature).
- Gradually ease into each stretch and hold for 5 to 10 seconds.
- Stretch to the point of gentle tension but not pain.
- Repeat each stretch at least two times.

Don't:

- Bounce, jerk, or force a stretch.
- Stretch to the point of pain.

Just prior to beginning the tests, all participants should be told to do the best they can on all tests but never to push themselves to a point of overexertion or beyond what they think is safe for them. Such a statement not only standardizes the testing instructions for all participants (these were the same directions given during the normative testing), but also helps clarify for the participants that the object on all test items is to try as hard as they *comfortably* can, while staying within their own safety limits.

Instructions to Participants

Participants should be encouraged to do the best they can on all tests, but never to push themselves to a point of overexertion or beyond what they think is safe for them.

Strict adherence to the points mentioned, as well as to the test protocols that follow, contributes not only to participant safety, but also to consistent and reliable testing procedures. Again, scores obtained from protocols that have been altered in any way or adapted to meet individual needs should *not* be compared to the normative standards, but can be used for individual evaluation from one testing time to another. The specific variation from the recommended protocols should be described in the comment section of the scorecard.

Official SFT Protocols

This section offers a full description of each of the SFT protocols. Included under each test item is its purpose, equipment requirements, test procedures, scoring instructions, and special safety and adaptation considerations. On each test item the instructor should first demonstrate the proper procedures at a reduced pace to assure that participants understand what is expected. Then, on each of the timed tests (chair stand, arm curl, 2-minute step, 8-foot up-and-go, and 6-minute walk), the demonstration should be repeated at a faster pace to illustrate that the objective is to do the best one can within safety limits.

CHAIR STAND TEST

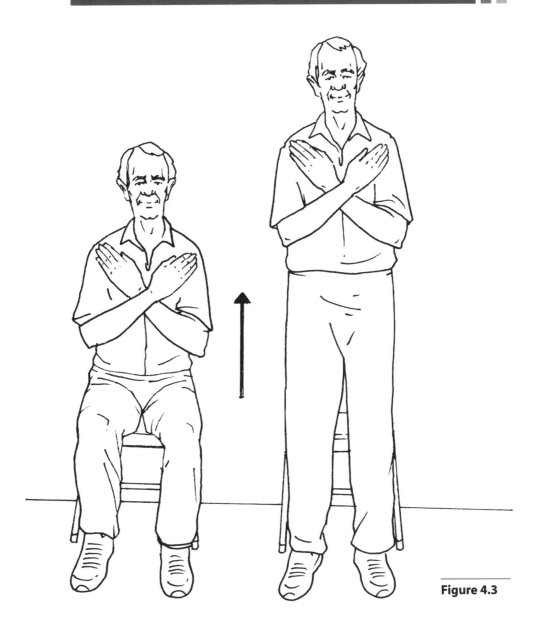

Figure 4.3

Purpose:

To assess lower-body strength

Equipment:

Stopwatch and straight-back or folding chair with a seat height of 17 in. (43.18 cm). Chair is placed against a wall to prevent slipping.

Procedure:

Instruct the participant to sit in the middle of the chair with back straight, feet flat on the floor, and arms crossed at the wrists and held against the chest. On the signal "go" the participant rises to a full stand, then returns to a fully seated position. See figure 4.3. Encourage the participant to complete as many full stands as possible in the 30 seconds. Demonstrate the test slowly to show proper form, then at a faster pace to show that the object is to do the best one can within safety

CHAIR STAND TEST *(continued)*

limits. Before testing, have the participant practice one or two stands to ensure proper form.

Scoring:

The score is the total number of stands completed in 30 seconds. If a person is more than halfway up at the end of 30 seconds, it counts as a full stand. Administer only one test trial.

Safety Tips:

- Brace the chair against the wall or have someone hold it steady.
- Watch for balance problems.
- Stop the test immediately if the participant complains of pain.

Adaptations:

If participants can't perform even one stand without using their hands, allow them to push off their legs or the chair, or use a cane or walker, if necessary. If an adaptation is needed, be sure to describe it on the scorecard. Although the recorded test score is zero for purposes of comparing to normative standards, also indicate the adapted score so that personal performance can be evaluated from one test time to the next.

ARM CURL TEST

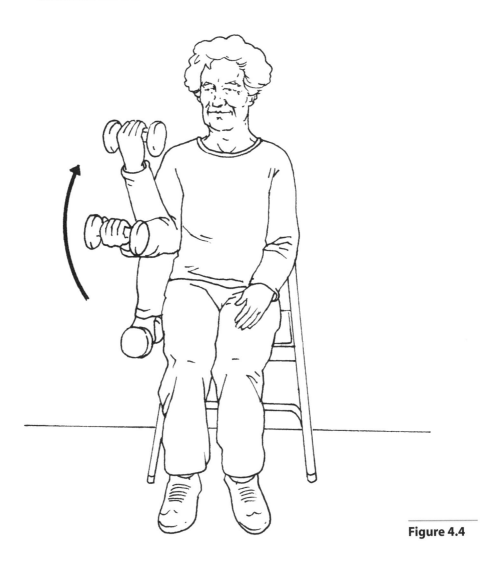

Figure 4.4

Purpose:
To measure upper-body strength

Equipment:
Stopwatch, straight-back or folding chair with no arms, 5-lb (2.27-kg) dumbbell for women, and 8-lb (3.63-kg) dumbbell for men

Procedure:
Have the participant sit on a chair with back straight and feet flat on the floor, and with the dominant side of the body close to the edge of the seat. The weight is held down at the side, perpendicular to the floor, in the dominant hand with a handshake grip. From the down position, the weight is curled up with the palm gradually rotating to a facing-up position during flexion. See figure 4.4. The weight is then returned to the fully extended down position with the handshake grip. Demonstrate the test slowly to illustrate the form, then at a faster speed to illustrate the pace. Have the participant practice one or two repetitions without the weight to ensure proper form.

ARM CURL TEST (continued)

On the signal "go" the participant curls the weight through the full range of motion (from full extension to full flexion) as many times as possible in 30 seconds. The upper arm must remain still throughout the test. Bracing the elbow against the body helps stabilize the upper arm.

Scoring:

The score is the total number of arm curls executed in the 30 seconds. If the arm is more than halfway up at the end of 30 seconds, it counts as a curl. Administer only one trial.

Safety Precautions:

Stop the test if the participant complains of pain.

Adaptations:

If a participant can't hold the hand weight because of some type of a health condition such as arthritis, a Velcro wrist weight can be used. If the weight is too heavy for the participant to complete even one repetition using the correct form, a lighter weight can be substituted. Record both the official test score (zero) and the adapted test score. Note the type of adaptation used to complete the test on the comment section of the scorecard.

6-MINUTE WALK TEST*

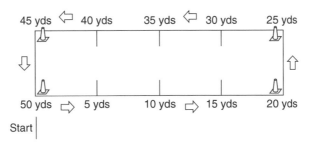

Figure 4.5

Purpose:

To assess aerobic endurance

Equipment:

Long measuring tape, two stopwatches, four cones (or similar markers), masking tape, magic marker, 12 to 15 popsicle sticks per person (or index cards and pencils to keep track of laps walked), chairs for waiting partners and for walkers who need to rest, and name tags

Setup:

Mark off in 5-yard segments a flat, 50-yard rectangular area (20 yards by 5 yards; see figure 4.5). The inside corners of the measured distance should be marked with cones, and the 5-yard lines marked with masking tape or chalk. (In metric units, this is a 45.7-meter course marked off in 4.57-meter segments.)

Procedure:

* Note: If the 6-minute walk test is selected as the aerobic endurance test, it should be administered after all other tests are completed.

Two or more participants should be tested at a time to standardize motivation. A skilled instructor can test up to 12 people at once, using partners to assist with scoring, but 6 at a time is more manageable. Starting (and stopping) times are staggered 10 seconds apart to encourage participants to walk at their own pace and not in clusters or pairs. Numbers (using name tags) are placed on participants to indicate the order for starting and stopping. On the signal "go" the participant begins walking as fast as possible (not running) around the course covering as much distance as possible in the 6-minute time limit. We recommend using two stopwatches to time the test, just in case one stops working. To keep track of the distance walked, partners give popsicle sticks (or similar objects) to participants each time they complete a lap. Or partners can mark a scorecard each time a lap is completed, using the "picket fence" system (𝍢𝍢 //, etc.).

The timer should move to the inside of the marked area after everyone has started. To assist with pacing, the remaining time should be called out when walkers are about half done, and when about 2 minutes are left. Participants can stop and rest on the chairs provided, but the time keeps running. The tester should encourage participants a few times by saying, "you're doing well" and "keep up the good work." When a participant's 6 minutes has elapsed, the tester asks him

6-MINUTE WALK TEST *(continued)*

or her to stop, move to the right (across from the nearest 5-yard marker), and slowly step in place for a minute to cool down.

Scoring:

Record the scores when all the walkers have been stopped. Each popsicle stick (or mark on a card) represents 50 yards. For example, if a person has 8 sticks (representing 8 laps) and was stopped next to the 45-yard marker, the score would be a total of 445 yards. Administer only one trial on test day. However, for improved pacing and maximum scoring accuracy, have participants practice a 6-minute walk on a day prior to test day.

Safety Precautions:

Select a well-lit walking area with a level, nonslip surface. Position chairs at several points along the outside of the walking area. Discontinue the test for any participant who shows signs of overexertion.

2-MINUTE STEP TEST

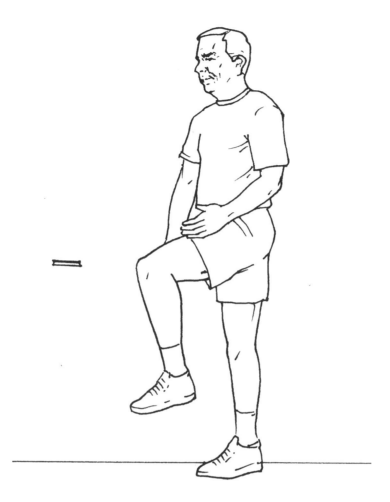

Figure 4.6

Purpose:

To provide an alternate test of aerobic endurance

Equipment:

Stopwatch, piece of string or cord about 30 in. (76.2 cm) long, masking tape, and a tally counter to help count steps

Setup:

Begin by setting the minimum knee-stepping height for each participant, which is at a level even with the midway point between the kneecap and the front hip bone (iliac crest). It can be determined using a tape measure or by simply stretching a piece of cord from the middle of the patella (kneecap) to the iliac crest, then folding it over and marking this point on the thigh with a piece of tape. See figure 4.6.

Monitoring Step Height:

You can monitor the correct knee height (stepping height) by moving the participant to the wall, a doorway, or next to a high-back chair and transferring the tape from the thigh to a spot at the same level on the wall or the chair. Step height also can be marked by stacking books on a nearby table.

2-MINUTE STEP TEST *(continued)*

Procedure:

On the signal "go" the participant begins stepping (not running) in place as many times as possible in the 2-minute period. Although both knees must be raised to the correct height, use your tally counter to count only the number of times the right knee reaches the target. When the proper knee height cannot be maintained, ask the participant to slow down, or to stop until he or she can regain the proper form, but keep the time running.

Scoring:

The score is the number of full steps completed in 2 minutes, that is, the number of times the right knee reaches the proper height. Administer only one trial on test day. However, for maximum scoring accuracy, have participants practice the test (stepping in place for 2 minutes) on a day prior to the test.

Safety Precautions:

Participants with balance problems should stand next to a wall, doorway, or chair (for support in case of lost balance) and should be spotted carefully. Monitor all participants closely for signs of overexertion. At the end of the test, ask participants to continue walking slowly for a minute to cool down.

Adaptations:

If participants are unable to lift their knees to the proper height or can lift only one to the proper height, allow them to complete the test, but indicate the change on the scorecard. If participants are unstable, they can hold onto a table, wall, or chair to complete the test. Note the type of adaptation used to complete the test on the comment section of the scorecard.

CHAIR SIT-AND-REACH TEST

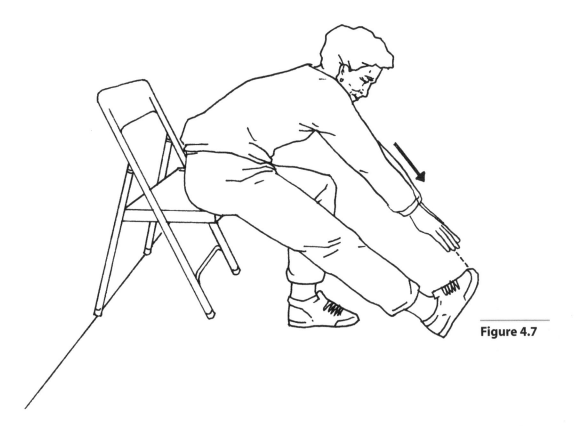

Figure 4.7

Purpose:
To assess lower-body (primarily hamstring) flexibility

Equipment:
Folding chair with a seat height of 17 in. (43.18 cm) and with legs that angle forward to prevent tipping, and an 18-in. (45.72-cm) ruler (half a yardstick)

Procedure:
The participant sits on the edge of the chair as shown in figure 4.7. The crease between the top of the leg and the buttocks should be even with the front edge of the chair seat. One leg is bent with the foot flat on the floor. The other leg is extended as straight as possible in front of the hip. The heel is placed on the floor, with the foot flexed at approximately 90 degrees.

With arms outstretched, hands overlapping, and middle fingers even, the participant slowly bends forward at the hip joint reaching as far forward as possible toward or past the toes. If the extended knee starts to bend, ask the participant to move slowly back until the knee is straight. The maximum reach must be held for two seconds.

The participant should practice the test on both legs to see which is preferred (the one resulting in the better score)*. Only the preferred leg is used for scoring purposes (for comparison to norms). Once the preferred leg is determined, have the participant practice a couple more times for warm-up.

---

*Although it is important to work on flexibility for both sides of the body, for the sake of time only the better side was used in establishing norms.

CHAIR SIT-AND-REACH TEST *(continued)*

Scoring:

After the participant has had two practice trials on the preferred leg, administer two test trials, record both scores, then circle the better one. Measure the distance from the tips of the middle fingers to the top of the shoe to the nearest half inch (centimeter). The midpoint at the top of the shoe represents the zero point. If the reach is short of this point, record the distance as a minus (-) score; if the middle fingers touch the toes, record a score of zero; and if the reach is past the midpoint of the toes, record the distance as a plus (+) score.

Safety Precautions:

Place the chair securely against a wall so it doesn't slip during testing. Remind participants to exhale as they bend slowly forward and to avoid bouncing. Participants should stretch only to a point of slight discomfort, never to the point of pain. Do not administer the test to people with severe osteoporosis or to those who have pain when flexing forward.

BACK SCRATCH TEST

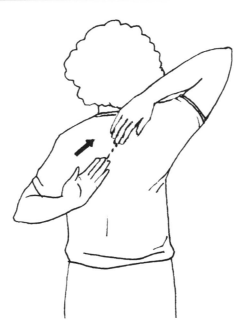

Figure 4.8

Purpose:
To assess upper-body (shoulder) flexibility

Equipment:
18-in. (45.72-cm) ruler

Procedure:
Have the participant stand and place his or her preferred hand over the same shoulder, palm down and fingers extended, reaching down the middle of the back as far as possible. See figure 4.8. Note that the elbow is pointed up. Ask the participant to place the other arm around the back of the waist with the palm up, reaching up the middle of the back as far as possible in an attempt to touch or overlap the extended middle fingers of both hands. The participant should practice the test to determine his or her preferred position (the hand over the shoulder that produces the best score)*. Two practice trials are given before scoring the test.

Check to see if the middle fingers are directed toward each other as best as possible. Without moving the participant's hands, direct the middle fingers to the best alignment. Do not allow participants to grab their fingers together and pull.

Scoring:
After giving the participant two warm-up practice trials in the preferred position, administer two test trials. Record both scores to the nearest half inch (cm), measuring the distance of overlap or distance between the tips of the middle fingers, then circle the better score. Give a minus (-) score if the middle fingers do not touch, a zero score if the middle fingers just barely touch, and a plus (+) score if the middle fingers overlap. Always measure the distance from the tip of one middle finger to the tip of the other, regardless of their alignment behind the back.

Safety Precautions:
Stop the test if the participant experiences pain. Remind participants to continue breathing as they stretch and to avoid any bouncing or rapid movements.

---

* Although it is important to work on flexibility for both sides of the body, for the sake of time only the preferred position was used in establishing norms.

8-FOOT UP-AND-GO TEST

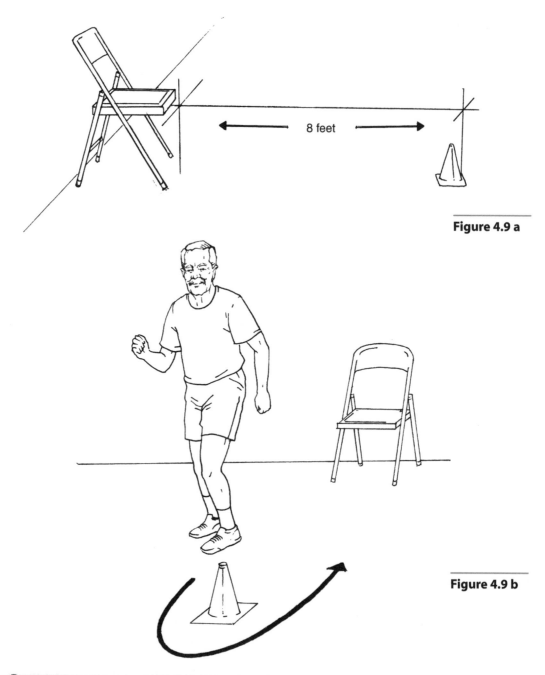

Figure 4.9 a

Figure 4.9 b

Purpose:
To assess agility and dynamic balance

Equipment:
Stopwatch, folding chair with 17-in. (43.18-cm) seat height, tape measure, and cone

Setup:
Place the chair against the wall facing a cone marker exactly 8 feet (2.44 meters) away, measured from the back of the cone to a point on the floor even with the front edge of the chair. See figure 4.9 a.

8-FOOT UP-AND-GO TEST

Procedure:

Instruct the participant to sit in the middle of the chair with back straight, feet flat on the floor, and hands on the thighs. One foot should be slightly in front of the other foot, with the torso slightly leaning forward. On the signal "go" the participant gets up from the chair, walks as quickly as possible around either side of the cone, and sits back down in the chair. See figure 4.9 b. Be sure to start the timer on the signal "go" whether or not the participant has started to move and stop the timer at the exact instant the person sits back down on the chair.

Scoring:

After you have demonstrated the proper form and desired pace, have the participant practice the test once and then administer two test trials. Record both times to the nearest tenth of a second, then circle the fastest time.

Safety Precautions:

When administering the 8-foot up-and-go test, stand between the chair and cone in order to assist participants in case they lose their balance. With the more frail person, watch that he or she stands up and sits down safely.

Adaptations:

If needed, a cane or walker can be used for this test, but scores should not be compared to the norms. Note on the comment section of the scorecard the type of adaptation used.

HEIGHT AND WEIGHT

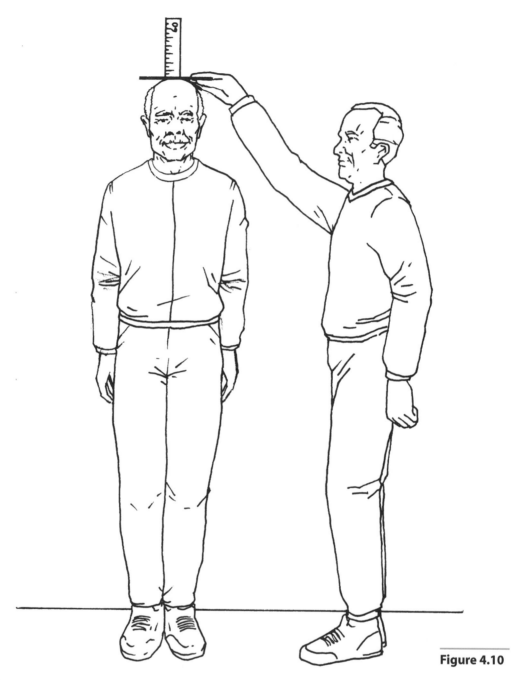

Figure 4.10

Purpose:

To assess body mass index (BMI)

Equipment:

Scale, 60-in. (152.4-cm) tape measure, masking tape, and ruler (or other flat object for marking the top of the head)

Procedure:

Shoes. For the sake of time, shoes can be left on during height and weight measurements, with adjustments made as described later.

HEIGHT AND WEIGHT

Height. Tape a 60-inch tape measure vertically on the wall with the zero end positioned exactly 20 inches up from the floor. Have the participant stand with the back of the head against the wall (the middle of the head is lined up with the tape measure) and the eyes looking straight ahead. Place a ruler (or similar object) on top of the participant's head, and while keeping it level, extend it straight back to the tape measure. See figure 4.10. The person's height is the score in inches indicated on the tape measure, plus 20 inches (the distance from the floor to the zero point on the tape measure). If shoes were worn, subtract one to two inches (or more) from the measured height, using your best judgment. Record height to the nearest half inch. (Note: A 60-inch tape measure is approximately equivalent to a metric tape of 150 cm. If a metric tape measure is used, for ease in calculating height, position it exactly 50 cm [equivalent to 19.7 in.] up from the floor. To adjust for shoe height, subtract two to four centimeters, using your best judgment. Record height to the nearest centimeter.)

Weight. Have the participant remove any heavy articles of clothing (jackets, heavy sweaters, etc.). Measure the person's weight and record it to the nearest pound (kilogram), with adjustments made for the weight of the person's shoes. In general, one pound (approximately half a kilogram) is subtracted for lightweight shoes and two pounds (approximately one kilogram) is subtracted for heavier shoes, using your best judgment.

Scoring:

Record the person's height and weight on the scorecard. You can estimate body mass index later using the height/weight conversion chart in appendix F. More precisely, you can determine BMI by dividing weight in kilograms by height in meters squared:

$$BMI = kg/m^2$$

or by multiplying the weight in pounds by 703, then dividing by the height in inches squared:

$$BMI = (lb \times 703)/in^2$$

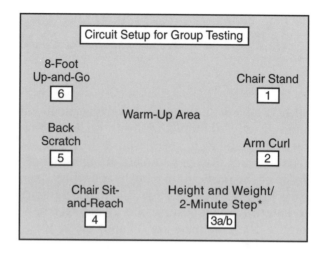

Figure 4.11 Order of station setup for group testing.

* If the 6-minute walk test is administered as the preferred test of aerobic endurance, the 2-minute step test is eliminated from station 3. The 6-minute walk test should always be administered last after all other tests are complete.

GUIDELINES FOR GROUP TESTING

It has been our experience that both practitioners and researchers generally find it preferable to administer the SFT to several people at a time. Although the SFT is especially suitable for group administration, careful preplanning and organization will be needed for the testing to run smoothly and efficiently. With the help of six to seven trained assistants, we have found that it is possible to test up to 24 participants at a time in a 60- to 90-minute time period using a circuit-style setup. If all tests, including the 6-minute walk test, are to be administered indoors, a large community center or gymnasium (approximately 50 feet by 100 feet or 15 meters by 30 meters) will be needed. However, a much smaller area will work if the 6-minute walk test can be administered outdoors or if the 2-minute step test is substituted for the 6-minute walk test as the measure of aerobic endurance. Included in this section are instructions for setting up the stations for testing, a list of equipment and supplies that will be needed at each station, guidelines for selecting and training testing assistants, and step-by-step procedures for administering the test items on test day.

Station Setup for Testing

For the most efficient use of time and to minimize the fatigue effect for participants, testing stations should be set up circuit-style in the following order: (1) chair stand test, (2) arm curl test, (3) height and weight and 2-minute step test (if 6-minute walk test is not used as the aerobic endurance test), (4) chair sit-and-reach test, (5) back scratch test, and (6) 8-foot up-and-go test. As indicated in the diagram in figure 4.11, the stations should be set up around the periphery of the room, allowing space in the center for the pretest warm-up exercises and for the 6-minute walk if there is room.

When the 6-minute walk test is used, it always should be administered after all other tests are completed. If it is not possible to give the 6-minute walk test (due to space limitations, bad weather, etc.), then the 2-minute step test is administered at station 3 along with the height and weight measurements. If you want to administer both the 2-minute step test and the 6-minute walk test, we recommend that the 2-minute step test be given as part of the regular circuit, with the 6-minute walk test administered on a separate day. For many older adults, it is too exhausting to complete both aerobic tests on the same day. Doing so could result in potentially unsafe conditions as well as inaccurate scoring.

For group testing, the specific procedures for administering each of the test items within the circuit is the same as that described in the preceding section under Official SFT Protocols. However, there will be a need for additional equipment and supplies, as well as for trained assistants to help at each of the stations.

Testing Equipment, Supplies, and Assistants

For group testing to run smoothly, each station should be properly set up in advance with all the required equipment and supplies. Although a special feature of the SFT is that it does not require extensive equipment, one should not underestimate how long it takes to round up the needed items. Table 4.2 lists the specific equipment and supplies, as well as the number of assistants, needed at each station. Brief organizational instructions are also provided. Recall that table 4.1 provides suggested vendors/sources for obtaining the equipment and supplies.

Although not absolutely necessary, it is convenient to have a small table (such as a card table) set up at each testing station, or, if possible, to arrange the testing stations near a counter, a table, a bench, or a ledge of some type that can provide a place to lay out the testing supplies (scorecards, pencils, stopwatches, etc.). To facilitate assigning and rotating participants, it also is helpful to post station signs indicating the test name and number of each station. Sample copies of station signs with brief test descriptions are included in appendix G. The signs can be copied, mounted, and laminated to make them more durable for repeated use.

As an aid in organizing and keeping track of all supplies and equipment, and in assuring that they are readily available at each station on test day, we have found it helpful to use numbered containers (e.g., gift bags or shopping bags) to collect and transport the items for each station. For example, a small bag labeled Station 1 would contain all of the items needed to conduct the chair stand test: a stopwatch, scorecards, and pencils. Similarly, a somewhat larger bag labeled Station 6 would contain the items needed for the 8-foot up-and-go: a stopwatch, tape measure, cone (or similar marker), scorecards, and pencils. In fact, if you plan to conduct the tests on multiple occasions, it is helpful to list the contents on the outside of each bag, making it easy to double-check to see that all equipment and supplies are available each time they are needed.

Selecting and Training Testing Assistants

For assessing groups of approximately 24 people at a time, resulting in four participants per station, a minimum of six to seven testing assistants will be required. If only three to four assistants are available, we suggest you limit your testing group to 12 instead of 24. Generally, one assistant is assigned to each station, with one exception. If the 2-minute step test is included at station 3 (meaning that it is given instead of the 6-minute walk test), then at least two, preferably three, assistants are needed at this station in order to maintain good timing and prevent a backlog in the timing of group rotations from one station to the next. If possible, the lead instructor or researcher should *not* be assigned to a testing station, but should be free to walk around to monitor the testing and help rotate groups, and

Table 4.2 Station Setup and Instructions for Testing up to 24 Participants at Once*

Station	Equipment	# of Testers	Brief Instructions
1. Chair stand test	Stopwatch	1	Demonstrate test; have all participants practice at once; test one at a time.
2. Arm curl test	Stopwatch 5-lb & 8-lb dumbbells (1 each)	1	Same instructions as station 1.
3. Height and weight; 2-minute step test	60-in. tape measure (mounted on wall) Two stopwatches, two tally counters, two 30-in. pieces of cord, masking tape	2[†]	Demonstrate step test to all; have all practice at once; each tester measures two people's height and weight and administers their step test.
4. Chair sit-and-reach test	18-in. ruler (half a yardstick)	1	Same instructions as station 1.
5. Back scratch test	18-in. ruler (half a yardstick)	1	Same instructions as station 1.
6. 8-foot up-and-go test	Stopwatch, cone, measuring tape	1	Demonstrate test; participants line up and take turns with practice test, trial one, and trial two.
All stations (1–6)	Each station needs four chairs for testing, or for resting while waiting for turn, four score cards, and four pencils.		
6-minute walk test	This test is given after all others, with all assistants helping. Equipment needs are described under Official SFT Protocols.		See 6-minute test protocol. An experienced tester can test 12 people at a time, with another 12 used as scoring partners; however, if time permits, testing 6 at a time works better.

* With 24 total participants, 4 are assigned to each station to begin testing, then are rotated clockwise through the 6-station circuit.

[†] Only one tester is needed at this station if the 6-minute walk test is given instead of the 2-minute step test.

to be available in an emergency situation. If additional assistants happen to be available to help with testing, by all means use them. Working in partnership during testing is more enjoyable for the assistants and has a positive effect on testing accuracy and efficiency.

Testing assistants can be older adult volunteers, co-workers, friends, and/or student volunteers from a nearby university. Active older adult volunteers are an especially ideal source of assistance provided they have good communication skills, as well as the physical and mental capabilities needed to demonstrate and conduct the tests properly. In fact, we have found older adults to be enthusiastic about helping with the tests, reliable, accurate, and even willing to go on the road to assist in testing at other locations, if needed. Regardless of the type of assistants you have, it is essential that they are properly trained and given ample time for practicing the tests before test day. All testers need to understand the exact procedures (protocols) for each test item and the importance of strictly following such procedures, or if necessary, of describing any deviation in proper protocol in the comment section of the scorecard. The following is a summary of the procedures that should be followed in training testing assistants.

- Provide all assistants with written descriptions and visual diagrams of the test protocols several days prior to testing and assign each assistant only one or two test items to learn and administer. The test descriptions in this chapter can be copied and distributed to test assistants.

- Ask the testing assistants to study their assigned test protocols and practice giving them to a friend or a family member.

- Schedule a testing practice day (rehearsal day) prior to the official test day for all assistants; demonstrate and review procedures for each of the test items.

- During the rehearsal, have the assistants practice giving their assigned tests to each other and check carefully for accuracy in testing and scoring.

- If you are including the 6-minute walk test as one of the test items, explain the protocol fully to your assistants during the practice day, emphasizing their role of helping to get all participants to the proper location for testing, helping to assign partners, watching for signs of overexertion during the test, and assisting with scoring at the end of the test. If time permits, assistants should partner up and practice the 6-minute walk test exactly as it will be given on test day.

Test Day Procedures

Based on our experience in administering the SFT to many different groups of older adults at numerous test sites, we have compiled the following list of test day procedures to help others with their planning. Following these steps should help your test day run smoothly.

1. You and all your assistants should arrive at the testing site at least 30 minutes prior to testing to set up the test stations and the 6-minute walk test course, if it is to be included.

2. Before participants arrive, call all test assistants together to review procedures and answer any last-minute questions.

3. Assign someone to collect all informed consent and medical clearance forms (if applicable) from participants.

4. After welcoming participants, you or an assistant should conduct a five- to eight-minute warm-up for the participants, including gentle stretching exercises. If possible, use lively music with the warm-up to promote enjoyment and a positive mood for the day.

5. Prior to sending participants to their stations, explain that the goal is to do the best they can on all tests but never to push themselves to a point of overexertion or beyond what they think is safe for them. Remind them that they should discontinue any activity that causes them pain or discomfort.

6. Following the warm-up and special instructions, direct the participants (in equal numbers) to one of the six stations. Have the participants remain at

their respective test stations until everyone has completed the test. Then ask participants to take their scorecards and rotate in a clockwise direction to the next station.

Sample testing scenario 1: Assuming 24 participants and six to eight assistants, four participants would be assigned to each of the six stations to begin the testing. Each assistant remains at the same station throughout the testing, while participants rotate from one station to the next.

Sample testing scenario 2: Assuming 12 participants and three to four assistants, four participants are assigned to stations 1, 3, and 5 to begin the testing. Each assistant then is responsible for conducting tests at two stations in a row. For example, when the assistant at station 1 completes the chair stand tests, he or she moves with these participants to station 2 to conduct the arm curl. Meanwhile, the assistants at station 3 also conduct the test at station 4, and so on. The participants eventually rotate to all six stations, while the assistants go back and forth between their two assigned stations.

7. If you have scheduled the 6-minute walk (which is always given after all other tests are completed), have participants bring their scorecards and walk together as a group to the test location. Refer to the 6-minute walk protocol described earlier in this chapter for setup and instructions. With a skilled instructor, it is possible to test up to 12 people at a time, using partners to help count laps. However, if time permits, testing 6 at a time is more manageable.

8. Following testing, collect all scorecards and thank participants for their cooperation and provide them with information as to when and how they will receive their test results.

SUMMARY

The SFT can be administered easily within the community setting. The complete test battery can be given to one or two people in about 30 minutes and, with the help of six or seven trained assistants, can be given to a group of up to 24 older adults in a 60- to 90-minute period. Important pretest considerations include the following:

- Properly training test technicians
- Obtaining informed consent
- Properly screening participants
- Providing pretest instructions to participants
- Gathering testing equipment and supplies
- Preparing scorecards
- Planning proper testing order
- Considering environmental conditions and signs of overexertion

On testing day it is important to include a proper warm-up, to provide standardized instructions to participants, and to conduct the tests according to the official SFT protocols described in this chapter. When deviations from proper protocols are necessary, they should be described in the comment section of the scorecard.

The SFT is especially conducive to group testing, but will require careful planning for the testing to run smoothly on test day. Specifically, special attention is needed with respect to (1) planning the testing circuit/stations, (2) gathering and organizing the equipment and supplies, (3) selecting and training testing assistants, and (4) planning the step-by-step testing day procedures.

Now that you know how to administer the SFT, the next chapter will provide information on interpreting the test results and providing feedback to clients. Suggestions will be made for using feedback to motivate clients and improve their performances.

5

TEST RESULTS

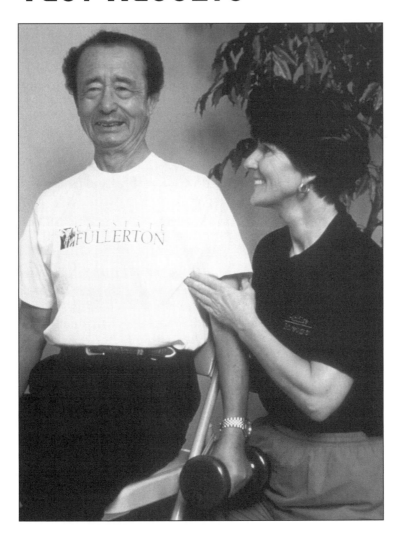

Interpreting and Using Feedback to Motivate and Improve Performance

We have found that after taking the Senior Fitness Test (SFT), most of the participants immediately want to know three things: what their scores are, what their scores mean, and how they can improve their scores. In this chapter we will explain how to interpret the results of the SFT items to your clients, including how to read the performance tables and charts that were developed as part of the national study to establish the fitness standards. We also will discuss ways of using the feedback from the test items to motivate your clients to increase their level of physical activity and improve their fitness level. Specifically, we will provide information on

- interpreting test scores,
- using test results to motivate participants, and
- improving physical performance.

INTERPRETING TEST SCORES

An important feature of the SFT is its accompanying performance standards that can be used in interpreting test results. As you will recall from chapter 3, performance standards can be either norm-referenced (standards that make it possible to compare one's scores to those of others of the same age and gender) or criterion-referenced (standards that represent a criterion behavior or goal, such as having the fitness level needed to perform everyday activities). Both normative and criterion-referenced standards were developed for the SFT based on a national study involving over 7,000 independent-living older adults, ages 60 to 94, from 267 different test sites throughout the United States. Data from the study were analyzed and then organized into various tables and charts that can be used in interpreting test scores.

Normative Tables

A common method of presenting normative data is through the use of percentile tables. Percentile norms indicate how a person's test scores rank relative to his or her peers. A percentile rank indicates the point in a distribution of scores below which that percentage of scores fall. For example, a chair stand test score of 15 for a 62-year-old woman falls at the 50th percentile (see the example in table 5.1), meaning that half (50%) of the women her age typically score below her and half score above her. However, another woman of the same age scoring 20 on the chair stand test would have a percentile rank of 90, indicating that she was better than 90% in her age group and that only 10% scored above her. Appendix H contains the percentile scores for women and men on each of the SFT items, making it possible for individuals in any of the five-year age groups to compare their scores to those of others of their same age and gender.

Percentile tables can also be used to compare a person's own scores across the different fitness categories. Determining the corresponding percentile rank for each fitness test score indicates an individual's relative strengths and weaknesses. For example, if a 73-year-old man obtained the following raw fitness scores, his corresponding percentile ranks (determined from appendix H) would tell us that he is above average in strength and endurance (at or near the 75th, 70th, and 90th percentiles), but below average (near the 20th percentile) in lower-body flexibility.

Table 5.1 Age Group Percentile Norms: Chair Stand Test (Women)

Percentile rank	60–64	65–69	70–74	75–79	80–84	85–89	90–94
95	21	19	19	19	18	17	16
90	20	18	18	17	17	15	15
85	19	17	17	16	16	14	13
80	18	16	16	16	15	14	12
75	17	16	15	15	14	13	11
70	17	15	15	14	13	12	11
65	16	15	14	14	13	12	10
60	16	14	14	13	12	11	9
55	15	14	13	13	12	11	9
50	15	14	13	12	11	10	8
45	14	13	12	12	11	10	7
40	14	13	12	12	10	9	7
35	13	12	11	11	10	9	6
30	12	12	11	11	9	8	5
25	12	11	10	10	9	8	4
20	11	11	10	9	8	7	4
15	10	10	9	9	7	6	3
10	9	9	8	8	6	5	1
5	8	8	7	6	4	4	0

Adapted from Rikli & Jones 1999.

Table 5.2 Example of Raw Scores and Percentile Equivalents

Test item	Raw score	Percentile rank (approximate) (for men ages 70-74)
Chair stand test (lower-body strength)	17	75th
Arm curl test (upper-body strength)	20	70th
6-minute walk test (aerobic endurance)	740	90th
Chair sit-and-reach test (lower-body flexibility)	–4.0	20th

Test results, such as those presented in table 5.2, can help in planning programs that are specifically targeted toward the needs of clients. Based on these test scores, a recommended exercise program for the gentleman in this example should include extra activities for improving his lower-body flexibility. Recording your client's percentile scores on a personal profile form, such as the one in figure 5.1, can help interpret personal strengths and weaknesses and track progress from one testing time to the next. The same form, in copy-ready format, is included in appendix I. Also, for those who have access to a computer, the *Senior Fitness Test*

Personal Profile Form

Name __John Doe__

Age __73__ M √ F __

Test Date: __2-12-01__

Test Item	Score	Rating* Below average ◄─ – – 25th%	Rating* Normal range – – – 75th%	Rating* Above average – – – ►	%ile rank[†]	Comments
Chair Stand (No. of stands)	17	—	√	—	75th	Keep up good work!
Arm Curl (No. of repetitions)	20	—	√	—	70th	Also good!
6-Minute Walk (yd) or **2- Minute Step** (steps)	740 yd	—	—	√	90th	Excellent! Keep up your walking program.
Chair Sit-&-Reach (No. of in. +/–)	–4.0	√	—	—	20th	Flexibility needs work. Add stretches for calf and hamstring muscles.
Back Scratch (No. of in. +/–)	–8.5	√	—	—	20th	Should add exercises for shoulder flexibility.
8-Foot Up-&-Go (No. of sec)	4.2	—	—	√	80th	Very good mobility.
Body Mass Index (See BMI chart)	Ht _67_ Wt _154_ BMI _24_	≤ 18 Underweight, may signify loss of muscle or bone 19–26 Healthy range ≥ 27 Overweight, may cause increased risk of disability/disease				

Figure 5.1   Sample personal profile form.

* Rating categories can be determined from tables 5.3 and 5.4 and are illustrated in the SFT performance charts (see figures 5.2 and 5.3).
† Percentile ranks are determined from tables in appendix H.

Software can be used to prepare personalized, professional-looking records for clients and can help maintain class records and document program outcomes.

Tables 5.3 and 5.4 provide an alternative version of the normative performance standards on each of the SFT items. Also see appendix M for a copy-ready version of these tables. In these simplified tables, only the normal range of scores is given

Table 5.3 Normal Range of Scores for Women*

	60–64	65–69	70–74	75–79	80–84	85–89	90–94
Chair stand test (# of stands)	12-17	11-16	10-15	10-15	9-14	8-13	4-11
Arm curl test (# of reps)	13-19	12-18	12-17	11-17	10-16	10-15	8-13
6-minute walk test** (# of yd)	545-660	500-635	480-615	435-585	385-540	340-510	275-440
2-minute step test (# of steps)	75-107	73-107	68-101	68-100	60-90	55-85	44-72
Chair sit-and-reach test† (in. +/–)	–0.5-+5.0	–0.5-+4.5	–1.0-+4.0	–1.5-+3.5	–2.0-+3.0	–2.5-+2.5	–4.5-+1.0
Back scratch test† (in. +/–)	–3.0-+1.5	–3.5-+1.5	–4.0-+1.0	–5.0-+0.5	–5.5-+0.0	–7.0--1.0	–8.0--1.0
8-foot up-and-go test (sec)	6.0-4.4	6.4-4.8	7.1-4.9	7.4-5.2	8.7-5.7	9.6-6.2	11.5-7.3

Table 5.4 Normal Range of Scores for Men*

	60–64	65–69	70–74	75–79	80–84	85–89	90–94
Chair stand test (# of stands)	14-19	12-18	12-17	11-17	10-15	8-14	7-12
Arm curl test (# of reps)	16-22	15-21	14-21	13-19	13-19	11-17	10-14
6-minute walk test** (# of yd)	610-735	560-700	545-680	470-640	445-605	380-570	305-500
2-minute step test (# of steps)	87-115	86-116	80-110	73-109	71-103	59-91	52-86
Chair sit-and-reach test† (in. +/–)	–2.5-+4.0	–3.0-+3.0	–3.0-+3.0	–4.0-+2.0	–5.5-+1.5	–5.5-+0.5	–6.5--0.5
Back scratch test† (in. +/–)	–6.5-+0.0	–7.5--1.0	–8.0--1.0	–9.0--2.0	–9.5--2.0	–9.5--3.0	–10.5--4.0
8-foot up-and-go test (sec)	5.6-3.8	5.9-4.3	6.2-4.4	7.2-4.6	7.6-5.2	8.9-5.5	10.0-6.2

* Normal range of scores is defined as the middle 50 percent of each age group. Scores above the range would be considered "above average" for the age group and those below the range would be "below average."

** Scores are rounded to the nearest five yards.

† Scores are rounded to the nearest half-inch.

for each age group, with *normal* defined as the middle 50% of the scores—that is, those falling between the 25th and 75th percentiles. To use these tables, you simply check to see whether a particular score falls within the normal range or if it is above or below the normal range. For a 72-year-old woman, a chair stand test score of 12 falls within the 10-15 range indicated for 70- to 74-year-olds and therefore would be evaluated as normal or typical for this age group. Chair stand test scores of 9 or lower, on the other hand, would be considered below normal for 70- to 74-year-olds, while scores falling above the indicated range (i.e., 16 or higher) would be considered above normal.

Criterion Performance Scores

Another way to evaluate test scores is to compare them to preset standards or reference points, such as the at-risk zones shown in figures 5.2 and 5.3. The data collected in our national study, in addition to providing information about what is typical for women and men at various ages, also provides information on fitness levels associated with high-functioning and low-functioning individuals. The average fitness scores for low-functioning women and men (i.e., for those in the study who reported having difficulty performing normal everyday activities such as climbing stairs, walking a half mile, or carrying groceries) provide a type of threshold value or criterion reference point that may signify being at risk for loss of functional mobility or functional independence. (See chapter 3 for additional details concerning the procedures for identifying the at-risk zones.)

Figures 5.2 and 5.3 provide graphical information showing normal, above normal, and below normal scoring ranges on each of the test items for women and men, as well as information on fitness levels that may place people at risk for losing their functional mobility. Figure 5.2a, for example, indicates that, regardless of age, a score below 8 on the chair stand test is associated with loss of functional mobility. Ideally, a person's goal would be not only to stay above the at-risk zone, but also to score far enough away from it so that he or she could withstand the usual age-related declines in performance and not reach the threshold associated with loss of function until very late in life.

Age, of course, is an important factor in interpreting one's score relative to being or becoming at risk for loss of functional mobility. Although a chair stand test score of 11 is above the at-risk zone for all age groups, it would be evaluated quite differently for a woman who is 82 years old compared to one who is 62. For an 82-year-old woman, a score of 11 would reflect normal lower-body strength—strength that would be unlikely to decline to the point of reaching the at-risk threshold during her lifetime assuming a normal rate of aging. For a 62-year-old woman, however, a score of 11, assuming a typical rate of decline (see the slope of the 25th percentile line in figure 5.2a), would place her at risk for loss of functional mobility by her late 70s. A 62-year-old woman who scores 14 or more chair stands, on the other hand, should be able to experience normal aging declines and not reach the at-risk zone until late in her 90s. The 25th and 75th percentile lines in figures 5.2 and 5.3 provide a general indication of the normal aging curves for each of the various test items. In appendix J, we have provided copy-ready charts of the information in figures 5.2 and 5.3, so you can copy and display them on a bulletin board.

Use the chart in appendix F to evaluate body mass index (BMI). Although an optimal BMI range for older adults has not been determined, a compilation of information from various sources suggests that BMI values above 26 or below 19 may be associated with increased risk for disease and disability in later years (American College of Sports Medicine, 1998b; Galanos et al., 1994; Harris et al.,

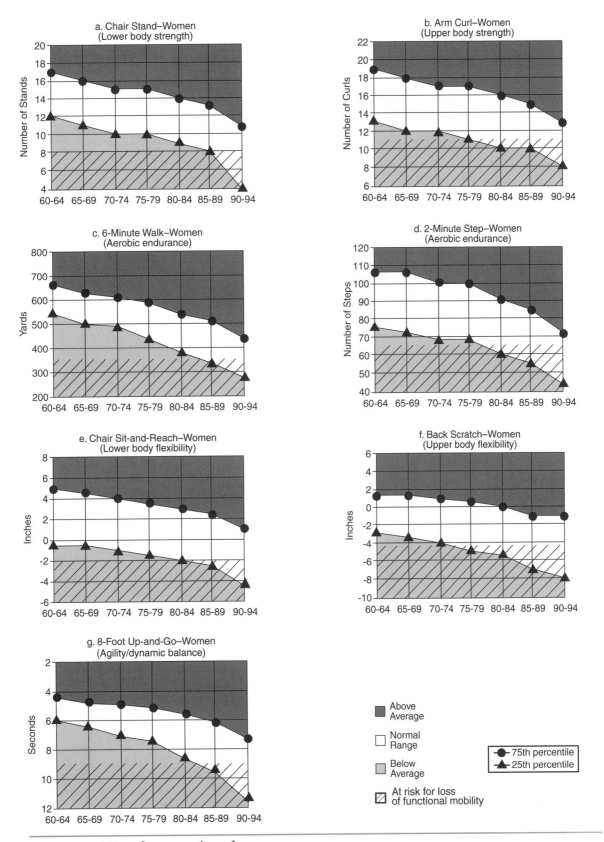

Figure 5.2 SFT performance charts for women.

Note: The at-risk zone boundaries were set based on the scores associated with low functional ability as reported in table 3.6. Values from the table are rounded to the nearest scoring unit.

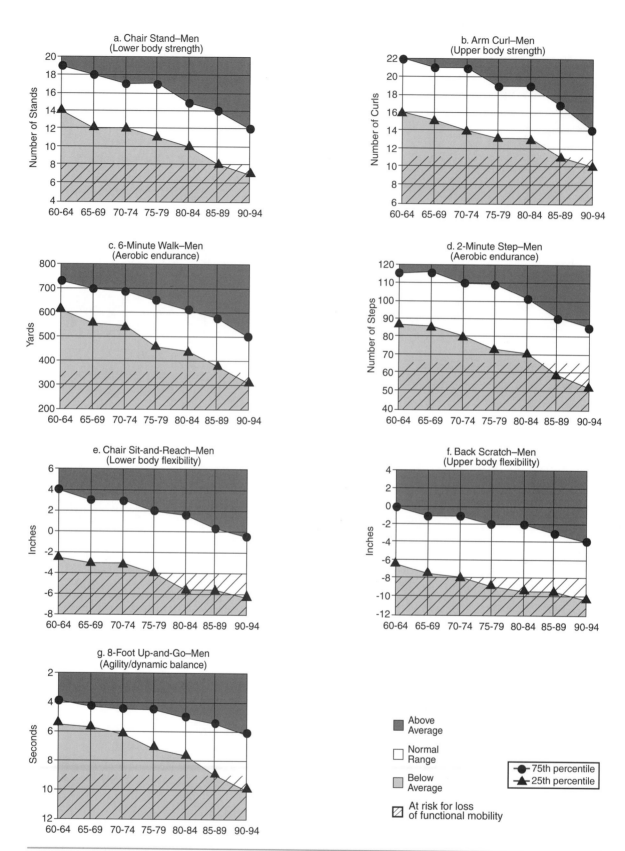

Figure 5.3 SFT performance charts for men.

Note: The at-risk zone boundaries were set based on the scores associated with low functional ability as reported in table 3.6. Values from the table are rounded to the nearest scoring unit.

1989; Losonczy et al., 1995; Shephard, 1997). Although BMI values provide useful body weight guidelines for most people, they should be interpreted with caution in older adults since unknown changes in bone and muscle loss can result in an increased chance of misclassification in this age group.

Precautions in Interpreting Scores

It is important to point out that the indicated at-risk zones in the SFT performance charts (figures 5.2 and 5.3) are based on our normative study only and should be thought of as general performance guidelines, rather than as absolute predictors of loss of function. Certainly, additional research is needed to validate these data. However, because of the large number of people tested in our study, we do think these data provide some useful, previously unavailable reference points (standards) for evaluating fitness levels in older adults.

Test users also are reminded that the threshold scores used to identify the at-risk zones represent group averages and may not apply equally to all individuals. For example, individuals who are very short (or perhaps very tall) may not have scored well on some of the test items due to their size, but may in fact be maintaining their functional ability quite well. Also, because these data are cross-sectional (collected across the different age groups at the same time) as opposed to longitudinal (collected on the same people as they progress through the aging process), the patterns of age-related declines illustrated in the charts could be under- or overestimations of the true rates of decline in most older people.

Further, in using the tables and charts to assist with interpretation of scores, it is important to keep in mind the overall characteristics of the normative population. As indicated in chapter 3, those participating in the study were independent-living volunteers who were fairly active, 89% Caucasian, and fairly well educated. Although the subject characteristics in the SFT study do not differ greatly from statistics reported for other large study populations of independent-living older Americans (see in chapter 3 the section titled Study Results/Participant Characteristics), it is important to note that the data in the tables represent *overall means* and may not be representative of individual subgroups of older adults. It is not clear, for example, how these scores would compare to different ethnic/racial groups, groups from other countries, groups with higher (or lower) levels of education, less motivated (nonvolunteer) participants, or individuals with multiple chronic health conditions.

Methods of Providing Feedback to Participants

Of the feedback mechanisms discussed earlier (tables, charts, personal profile forms, or computerized printouts), the ones that will work best for explaining test results to your participants will depend on several factors. If you have given the SFT to a large group and have little time to provide individualized feedback, it will probably work best for you to return the individual scorecards to participants (after you've made copies) and let them compare their scores to standards that have been posted, using either the normal range of scores tables (appendix M) or the SFT performance charts (appendix J). By referring to the charts, participants can compare their scores with those of other people their age and will find out whether their performance on each test would be considered normal, above normal, below normal, or at risk for their age group. Before giving back the scorecards, we recommend that you meet with your group to explain what the norms represent, how to use the tables and charts, and especially what can be done to improve performance for those who score low.

If time and resources permit, however, more meaningful feedback can be provided to clients through the use of individualized personal profile forms, either the hand-prepared version in appendix I or the printout generated from the *Senior Fitness Test Software*. These forms provide clients with the information they need to interpret their scores. Raw scores are listed for each test item along with the corresponding percentile ranks, the evaluation category (normal, above normal, below normal, or at risk), and personalized comments and suggestions if appropriate. Using these forms makes it easy to evaluate a person's relative strengths and weaknesses within the fitness categories (i.e., what the client is best or worst at) and makes it easy to compare scores from one testing time to the next. In the computerized version, the software program evaluates each individual's scores relative to the established standards and provides clients with easy-to-read charts explaining their scores. The computer software also facilitates ongoing record-keeping of your clients and provides you with handy group statistics for evaluating the effectiveness of your total program.

Again, regardless of the feedback method used, remember that it is critically important for you to help clients understand that *no matter what their age or current condition, improvement is always possible!* Never just assess clients and give them feedback about their fitness, especially if their scores are low, without giving them hope and encouragement at the same time. Instead, explain to them that numerous studies have shown that it is never too late and that people are never too old to improve their fitness, and that you will help them plan exercise activities to improve their performance if they so desire. We also suggest that you help clients to understand that although the normative standards (charts) make it possible for them to compare their scores with those of others their age, the more important concern is how their own scores change over time. This is especially important for people with low performance scores so that they won't become discouraged. Suggestions for motivating participants to increase their physical activity level and improve their performance are discussed in the next section.

USING TEST RESULTS TO MOTIVATE PARTICIPANTS

Almost everyone recognizes that adequate physical activity is important for optimum health and functioning, yet few people (less than 20% of older adults) get the amount of activity they need. According to exercise experts, an important first step in motivating people to become more active is to assess their fitness level and provide individualized feedback, presuming, of course, that people are at the stage of at least contemplating becoming more active. In fact, Dr. Kenneth Cooper, the founder and medical director of the world-renowned Cooper's Aerobic Center in Dallas, designed his entire program based on the premise that evaluation is the most powerful motivator for getting people to improve their fitness level (Cooper, 1995). According to Cooper, and according to our own experiences in working with older adults, the steps to success in getting people to change their activity behaviors are:

- *Evaluation*—assessing people's current level of fitness, identifying strengths and weaknesses;
- *Education and motivation*—helping people understand why fitness is important in their lives;

- *Goal-setting and program planning*—planning and carrying out a relevant program based on individual goals, one designed to meet individual needs and interests; and

- *Monitoring progress and reevaluation*—checking participants' progress and adjusting the program as needed.

If you have given the SFT to your clients, you already have completed the first of these steps, that of evaluation. For many individuals, simply having their fitness level assessed motivates them to increase their activity level and improve their fitness. Procedures for addressing the steps subsequent to evaluation are described in the following paragraphs.

Educating and Motivating Participants

After administering the SFT to your clients/program participants, we suggest that you meet with them, either individually or as a group, to give them their feedback. This provides an ideal time to educate and motivate them about the importance of being physically active and fit in later years. You especially should point out the strong relationship between people's activity level and their fitness scores (surprisingly, many people are not aware of this) and the fact that at least half of the typical decline associated with aging is not due to aging at all, but rather to disuse—that is, people's tendency to become less and less active as they age.

Point out to your clients that as people are living longer, it is becoming increasingly important that they pay attention to their fitness level if they want to remain healthy and independent during their later years. Communicating how participation in physical activity can help to delay the onset of physical frailty and extend people's physical independence can be very motivating. Statistics indicate that many older adults by their late 70s or early 80s, particularly those with sedentary lifestyles, will lose the strength and endurance they need to perform common everyday activities such as climbing stairs, walking to the store, and taking care of their own personal and household activities, unless steps are taken to increase their activity level. For many, maintaining a physically active lifestyle can easily add 10 to 15 years or more to their functional or active life span, thus significantly delaying the onset of physical frailty.

It is especially critical for older people to understand the importance of preventing the vicious cycle that occurs for so many—the cycle that begins with people becoming less active as they age, which in turn leads to lower energy levels (less desire to want to be active), which then results in even further reductions in activity, then further declines in energy level, and on and on. Eventually, this downward spiral can result in people's strength and endurance declining to the point at which it is hazardous to their health and ability to carry out normal everyday activities. Scores obtained on the SFT items can provide important feedback about the strengths and weaknesses of older adults and whether or not their rate of physical decline is placing them at risk for losing their functional mobility.

The good news that you can share with your clients, however, is that no matter what their age or current physical condition, it is always possible to improve their level of fitness by increasing their activity level. You can tell them, citing research conducted at Tufts University, Cal State Fullerton, San Diego State University, and elsewhere, that people of all ages—even into their late 80s and 90s—have experienced significant gains in fitness after beginning exercise programs, gains that have led to improved functional performance (walking and balance, for example) and, for some, the ability to discard their canes and walk without assistance (Boyd

& Zizzi, 1999; Fiatarone et al., 1990; Fiatarone et al., 1994; Rikli & Edwards, 1991; Rose, Jones, Dickin, Lemon, & Bories, 1999; Verfaillie, Nichols, Turkel, & Hovell, 1997).

You can also motivate your clients by sharing success stories from your own program. Older people are interested in the activities of their peers and are often motivated by their successes. In our program, for example, a 79-year-old woman who had several chronic health conditions and was on 13 medications, scored in the at-risk area on most test items when she came in to be tested. She was so surprised at how poorly she scored compared to others her age that she immediately hired a personal trainer. Six months later, when she came back for a reevaluation, she not only scored in the normal range on all tests, but she was down to taking only four medications and said she felt like a new person. She also looked like a new person—full of energy and smiles. Certainly we are not suggesting that exercise is the answer to curing medical problems, but we do know that it can help in managing numerous conditions.

> *"Since I have been exercising, I have noticed positive changes in balance, flexibility, and endurance. The annual tests (Senior Fitness Tests) allow me to track my improvements. I believe that because of my exercise program, my overall physical conditioning has improved, as well as an old knee injury that has steadily gotten better."*
>
> **George Schussler, age 75—**
> **Maple Knoll Wellness Center (Cincinnati, Ohio)**

Even relatively small success stories can be interesting and meaningful. One woman, after eight weeks in our program, was thrilled when she found that she had gained enough upper-body strength to be able, for the first time, to pull down the back door (hatch) in her minivan without having to ask for help. Another woman reported a tremendous gain in self-confidence when her lower-body strength (and balance) improved to the point at which she could get up from the floor easily without help, something she had been unable to do for some time. We could go on and on with stories about how increased physical activity level has improved people's quality of life.

Beginning or modifying an exercise program, however, generally takes more than a motivational talk about the value of exercise and a few motivational stories. Changing behavior in people is difficult and almost always requires applying some type of behavior modification strategy. One behavior modification technique that has been successful in changing exercise behavior, especially for those who already have expressed a desire to change, is that of goal-setting.

Goal-Setting and Program Planning

Goal-setting is an essential step for anyone wanting to make a change in behavior. Establishing goals, especially written goals, tends to move people from a good-intentions or wishful-thinking level to an action-plan level. As an exercise leader, you should encourage your clients to participate in goal-setting, but you should *not* set their goals for them. People are much more likely to work toward the goals *they* think are important, rather than goals that have been established by others, including those established by noted professional groups such as the American College of Sports Medicine or the U.S. surgeon general (unless, of course, these can be personalized and seen as important to them as individuals). In helping your clients with goal-setting, the following procedures and considerations may be helpful. Specifically, you should encourage your clients to do the following:

1. **Identify long-term goals or major exercise objectives.** You can expect that there will be great variation in what people hope to accomplish in their exercise programs. Some may be interested in addressing a specific weakness that was identified in their SFT results, while others may just want to maintain their current mobility and energy level. Others may be interested in managing a health condition (reducing their blood pressure, controlling their diabetes, etc.). Some may want to lose weight, improve their appearance, or reduce their risk of falling. Still others may want to improve their performance in a particular sport, such as golf or running. Also, some people's goals may be very specific, such as losing 10 pounds before a granddaughter's wedding the following summer, whereas others may be more general. For the goal-setting process to be most effective, goals should be recorded in writing, perhaps using a form similar to the one in appendix K.

2. **Identify short-term goals (one- or two-week activity plans).** Long-term goals are more likely to be attained if broken down into more immediate short-term goals. Short-term goals should be realistic, measurable, time-specific, and should not extend beyond one or two weeks. They should be expressed as specific activities that clients think will move them toward their long-term goals. Some suggest that a goal is realistic only if it meets the 90% rule—that is, it is one that the client is 90% sure of being able to achieve within the time period stated. A measurable goal (or activity) is one that is observable. A goal of exercising more is not observable, but a goal of increasing one's walking time to at least 30 minutes a day at least four times a week is observable. Being time-specific relative to one's goals means planning the days and times that the activity will take place, such as walking every Monday, Wednesday, and Friday morning at 9:00, or performing 10 minutes of stretching exercises each evening during the 6 o'clock news. Scheduling activity into one's day/week (i.e., putting it on the calendar) increases the likelihood that it will occur. Short-term goals (action plans) and timetables should be recorded on the client's goal-setting form along with long-term goals (see appendix K).

3. **Identify potential obstacles and plan strategies for overcoming them.** Recognizing that there will be obstacles and setbacks in carrying out one's activity goals, it is important to try to predict in advance what these might be and plan possible strategies for dealing with them. Most people can predict what the most likely obstacles will be for them. It may be bad weather, interruptions from friends or relatives, or simply a lack of self-discipline. If weather frequently interrupts walking plans, perhaps back-up plans can be made for going to the mall or to a fitness center on bad-weather days. If procrastination or lack of self-discipline is a major barrier, it may help to schedule exercise sessions with a partner. The extra social pressure and expectations from partners, as well as the added enjoyment of exercising together, can help people stay on target with their plans. Projected obstacles and the strategies for overcoming them should be spelled out clearly as part of the goal-setting process (see appendix K).

Monitoring Progress and Reevaluation

Another important step in changing physical activity behavior is that of monitoring progress and reevaluating. To promote program adherence, you might suggest to your clients that they discuss their goals/plans with a friend, a family member, or with you as their instructor and then ask this person to sign their goals contract as a witness to their plans. They might even ask their witness to question them about their progress at least once a week.

For some people, it also can be motivating to keep a daily or weekly exercise log to track and record their progress toward their long-term goals (such as losing 10 pounds) and to monitor their adherence to weekly activity plans. In fact, it is important to recognize that increasing one's activity level is a worthy accomplishment by itself and often leads to other unexpected rewards (apart from the original goal) such as feeling and looking better, improved self-confidence or self-efficacy, sleeping better, or having a higher level of energy and ambition. Interestingly, these supplemental, more intrinsic rewards are often most responsible for keeping people active long after their original goal has been met (the 10 pounds have been lost and the granddaughter's wedding is over).

The challenging part, however, is that it takes time (sometimes many weeks) for a person to reach the stage at which the intrinsic rewards associated with physical activity and fitness (e.g., the joy of being active, the sense of well-being, and the feeling of accomplishment) become sufficient motivation for maintaining an exercise program. In the meantime, you should encourage your clients, especially your new clients, to continue with the goal-setting activities described earlier, and also to consider keeping an exercise log of their activities. Figure 5.4 contains an example of a fairly generic weekly activity chart that should be adaptable for most people. Although people's exercise goals and plans may vary considerably, most will be best served by planning activities in the general categories indicated. Appendix L contains a copy-ready form of this chart.

Progress toward one's goals should also be monitored through periodic re-evaluation of fitness parameters and other relevant indicators. Readministering the SFT after several weeks provides an indication of progress with respect to changes in strength, endurance, flexibility, agility and balance, and body weight. Changes in other indicators such as blood pressure, blood sugar readings (if diabetic), golf scores, or self-diagnosed energy level and feelings of well-being also provide evidence of progress toward goals.

As clients are setting their goals and planning their programs, they may ask you for guidance in helping them determine what specific activities will best help them reach their goals. The next section addresses a number of relevant considerations in helping your clients improve their performance.

IMPROVING PERFORMANCE

In recommending specific exercises to help your clients improve their fitness, several factors should be taken into account. In addition to considering their current fitness needs as indicated by their SFT scores, as well as any personal exercise objectives they have (such as losing weight or managing a health condition), it also is important to consider clients' exercise/activity preferences. We often hear that the best exercise to improve performance is the one that people will do, suggesting that you also should help your clients determine which types of exercise options are most likely to work for them—that is, which ones best fit their personalities and meet other personal and environmental needs (e.g., access to facilities, financial considerations, transportation, social support, etc.). Various exercise options can include exercising alone versus in groups; exercising at home versus going to an exercise class or a fitness center; engaging in structured exercise

Activity Record

Week of _____

Name _____

Record # of minutes per day	Sunday	Monday	Tuesday	Wednesday	Thursday	Friday	Saturday
Lifestyle activity: Indicate any moderately strenuous housework, yard work, recreation, sports, etc. If low active, should add structured exercise (see below).		Cleaned patio, some yard work (30 min)					Cleaned house (vacuumed, mirrors, baths, etc.) 1 1/2 hrs.
Structured Exercise: *Aerobic exercise*—brisk walking, jogging, aerobic exercise, cycling, treadmill, etc. (Need 20-30 min 3-5 times a week.)		Brisk walk (30 min)		Brisk walk (30 min)		Rode cycle at Senior Center (20 min)	
Strengthening exercise—can use elastic band/tubing, hand weights, weight machines, or calisthenics. (Work upper and lower muscles at least 2 times a week.)			20 min upper & lower body		20 min (upper & lower)		Housework (see above)
Daily totals: Are you getting 30-40 min of moderate exercise on most days?		60 min	20 min	30 min	20 min	20 min	90 min
Also important: *Flexibility/stretching*—should stretch all muscle/joint areas 2-3 times a week, preferrably daily.		Lots of stretching after walking				Flexibility & relaxation exercises before bedtime.	
Agility/balance activities—especially important for those experiencing loss of balance.							

Figure 5.4 Sample activity record.

activities versus incorporating exercise into daily routines; or developing an active hobby, doing more yard work or housework, or getting one's exercise through various recreational, social, dance, or sport activities. In helping clients plan effective exercise programs, it also is important to consider the scientifically-documented exercise guidelines and recommendations that have been developed by professional experts.

In the remaining sections of this chapter, we will review the recently published exercise guidelines that apply to older adults and make exercise recommendations relative to improving performance. Our recommendations will include ways of increasing lifestyle physical activity, as well as structured exercises that address specific fitness categories.

Exercise Guidelines for Older Adults

Several recent reports, particularly the surgeon general's report (SGR), *Physical Activity and Health* (U.S. Department of Health and Human Services, 1996); the American College of Sports Medicine's (ACSM) Position Stand on Exercise and Physical Activity for Older Adults (American College of Sports Medicine, 1998a); and the most recent ACSM *Guidelines for Exercise Testing and Prescription* (American College of Sports Medicine, 2000) have provided us with sound, data-based guidelines for making exercise recommendations for older adults. The surgeon general's report, based on over 1,000 scientific studies from the fields of epidemiology, exercise science, medicine, and the behavioral sciences, suggests that older adults can experience both health and functional mobility benefits from engaging in a moderate level of physical exercise on most, preferably all, days of the week.

For most older adults, moderate exercise (defined as that which burns at least 150 calories of energy per day or about 1,000 calories a week) would be something equivalent to 30 to 40 minutes of brisk walking per day. Table 5.5 lists examples of other activities providing moderate amounts of exercise. The SGR also indicates that additional benefits can be gained from engaging in even greater amounts of physical activity, with the increased activity being spread over the day as part of one's normal daily activities or occurring as a result of increased participation in structured exercises. Finally, recognizing that muscular strength is so critical to functional mobility, the SGR also suggests that at least some of an older adult's physical activity program should consist of strengthening exercises.

ACSM's exercise guidelines for older adults (American College of Sports Medicine, 1998a, 2000) are consistent with the recommendations of the surgeon general's report, but include additional details. Specifically, they provide evidence suggesting that for optimal health and functioning in later years, older adults should engage in (1) moderate aerobic exercise on most days of the week—exercise that involves large-muscle rhythmic activities such as walking, running, swimming, or cycling; (2) strengthening activities at least twice a week, including relatively high-intensity, progressive resistance exercises if the goal is to increase muscular strength; and (3) activities that improve flexibility, balance, and agility. It is important to note that frail, low-fit individuals may need to engage in gradual strengthening exercises to improve their muscular fitness *before* they can begin an aerobic exercise program. In frail older adults, improvements in walking ability, for example, generally will depend on improvements in lower-body strength and balance.

Although a well-rounded program for older adults should address each of these fitness categories (aerobic endurance, strength, flexibility, and balance/agility), there are many options for getting the recommended amount of exercise. Even

Table 5.5   Examples of Activities That Provide Moderate-Level Exercise

Exercises that use 150 calories of energy
• Washing and waxing a car for 45 to 60 minutes
• Washing windows or floors for 45 to 60 minutes
• Gardening for 30 to 45 minutes
• Pushing self in a wheelchair for 30 to 40 minutes
• Walking 1 3/4 miles in 35 minutes (20 min/mile)
• Walking 2 miles in 30 minutes (15 min/mile)
• Raking leaves for 30 minutes
• Pushing a stroller 1 1/2 miles in 30 minutes
• Bicycling 5 miles in 30 minutes
• Bicycling 4 miles in 15 minutes
• Doing water aerobics for 30 minutes
• Swimming laps for 20 minutes
• Running 1 1/2 miles in 15 minutes (10 min/mile)
• Stair walking for 15 minutes
• Social dancing for 30 minutes
• Shoveling snow for 15 minutes

though it is beyond the scope of this book to provide a full discussion of exercise programming for older adults, we will make a few recommendations and provide a list of resources where additional information can be found.

Exercise Recommendations

Again, in recommending specific exercises for people, it is important to keep in mind that the only ones that will be effective will be the ones that they will do! With that in mind, we recommend that you explain to your clients that they can improve their fitness level in two ways: (1) by incorporating additional physical activity into their normal daily routines (sometimes referred to as lifestyle exercise) or (2) by scheduling time each week to engage in structured types of exercises designed to address specific fitness components, such as strength, endurance, and flexibility. Each of these methods has advantages. For some, the advantage of lifestyle exercise is that it also has other purposes (e.g., walking the dog, doing yard work, or washing the car) and doesn't seem like *real* exercise. The advantage of structured exercise is that it focuses on specific aspects of fitness and is especially effective in addressing any special needs or weaknesses that may have been identified during the client's fitness assessments. The following sections offer additional suggestions of lifestyle exercise and structured exercise.

Lifestyle Exercise

Most people could significantly increase their activity level and improve their fitness simply by building more activity into their daily lives. Every day there are numerous opportunities to become more active just by altering our normal routines and habits—by taking the stairs instead of the elevator, by walking more and driving less, and by doing more house and yard work, as examples. We especially suggest that you try to instill in your older clients the idea that "moving more and sitting less" is good for them. Considering that the use-it-or-lose-it phenomenon becomes increasingly more real as we age, the best thing we can do to assure continued functional ability is to continue to stay as active as possible. The following are just a few examples of how people could significantly increase their daily energy expenditures:

- Take the stairs instead of an elevator or escalator.
- Walk the dog more often.
- Walk to the store instead of driving.
- Bicycle to a friend's house.
- Clean the garage or car.
- Do more housework and yard work.
- Play with your grandchildren.
- Join a hiking club or dance group.
- Volunteer for active projects.
- Park farther away.
- Plan active vacations.
- Pull a golf cart instead of riding.
- Take up an active hobby.
- Pick up litter in public places (parks, beaches, etc.).

These lifestyle activities can help maintain functional ability and fitness, and may even result in significant increases in fitness levels if there is a substantial increase in activity expenditure over what a person has been accustomed to. For most people, however, additional benefits can be gained from supplementing their lifestyle activity with a structured exercise program that specifically addresses each of the major fitness categories.

Structured Exercises

In addition to incorporating as much activity as possible into their daily routines, (i.e., moving more and sitting less), most older adults also could benefit from setting aside time each day for specific strength, aerobic, or flexibility exercises, thus assuring a well-rounded program of activities that addresses all aspects of fitness. Structured or focused exercise is especially important for clients who received low scores on the SFT and need to improve their fitness in one or two specific categories. The following information on exercise is specific to each of the major components of fitness—aerobic endurance, strength, flexibility, and balance and agility.

Aerobic Endurance. Aerobic exercise improves the function of the heart, lungs, and blood vessels and helps people have more energy. In the SFT aerobic endurance is measured using either the 6-minute walk test or the 2-minute step test. Your clients can best improve their aerobic endurance scores by engaging in large-muscle rhythmic activities such as walking, jogging, swimming, or cycling. For people whose aerobic endurance scores were exceptionally low on the SFT, we suggest they work on their lower-body strength (see the next section) to improve it before, or at the same time as, working to improve their aerobic endurance. For most older adults, walking is an ideal form of aerobic exercise, not only because it contributes to one's aerobic fitness, but also because of its importance in everyday functioning.

The goal of aerobic conditioning is to gradually increase the exercise duration, frequency, and intensity to the point at which one can maintain the activity for 30 to 40 minutes at a time, preferably at least five times a week, at a moderate level of intensity. For most, a moderate intensity level would be that which causes a noticeable increase in breathing rate and heart rate and usually results in some amount of perspiration. Some use the "talk test" to define moderate intensity exercise, meaning that when exercising at a moderate level, people should still be able to talk, but not sing. Another way of determining moderate intensity level is through the use of Borg's Rate of Perceived Exertion (RPE) scale presented in table 5.6. On the RPE scale, moderate exercise is defined as that with an intensity level of 12 to 14, that is, exercise that would be evaluated as being in the "somewhat hard" range.

As with all types of exercise, you should always advise your clients to start slowly and work up gradually to the desired level. Studies show that aerobic exercise is equally effective if performed in continuous bouts (such as 30 minutes at one time) or in shorter bouts (such as 10 minutes at a time, three times a day). The amount (duration) of aerobic exercise needed to meet the guidelines recommended by the surgeon general and by the ACSM varies depending on the intensity level. Table 5.5 contains examples of activities that provide the recommended amounts of daily moderate-level physical activity—that is, activities that use approximately 150 calories of energy per day or 1,000 calories per week, assuming daily participation (U.S. Department of Health and Human Services, 1996). Increased participation in these types of aerobic activities should result in improved performance on the SFT aerobic endurance tests: the 6-minute walk and the 2-minute step tests.

Table 5.6   Borg's Rate of Perceived Exertion Scale (RPE)

6	No exertion at all
7	Extremely light
8	
9	Very light
10	
11	Light
12	
13	Somewhat hard
14	
15	Hard
16	
17	Very hard
18	
19	Extremely hard
20	Maximal exertion

Reprinted from Borg 1998.

Aerobic Conditioning Guidelines

- Choose large-muscle rhythmic activities such as walking, jogging, cycling, swimming, or aerobic dancing.
- Exercise on most, preferably all, days of the week.
- Start slowly, but work up to at least 30 to 40 minutes of aerobic activity each day.
- Exercise at a moderate (somewhat hard) level of intensity.

Muscular Strength. As discussed in chapters 2 and 3, maintaining an adequate amount of lower- and upper-body strength is necessary for executing a variety of common tasks such as climbing stairs, walking distances, getting out of a chair or the bathtub, and lifting and carrying objects. In the SFT, lower-body strength was assessed using a chair stand test. Upper-body strength was measured using an arm (bicep) curl test. Any form of exercise that stresses a person's muscles, including many common types of housework and yard work activities, will help in maintaining strength. However, if your client scored low on one or both of the SFT strength items and wants to increase his or her strength, a particular regimen of progressive resistance exercises will need to be followed.

Briefly, strength is increased by gradually increasing the resistance placed on a muscle, that is, by applying what is called the overload principle. Overloading a muscle means making it do more than it is accustomed to doing. This can be accomplished using free weights (similar to the dumbbells used to test arm strength in the SFT), elastic exercise bands, Velcro strap-on weights, exercise machines that are designed for specific muscle groups, or a person's own body weight and gravity.

A recommended procedure for increasing strength in older adults involves performing 10 to 15 repetitions of a particular strengthening exercise using a weight (resistance) that would cause the muscles to fatigue within the 10 to 15 repetitions, with *fatigue* meaning that the muscles cannot perform another repetition using proper form. Using the bicep curl as an example, bicep strength can be increased by selecting a hand weight (dumbbell) that can be curled at least 10 times, but no more than 15 times, before the muscle is too fatigued to continue. Then, as muscle strength improves (as it becomes possible to curl the selected weight more than 15 times before fatigue), the size of the weight is increased, causing the muscle to again be overloaded—to do more than it was accustomed to. This process is repeated throughout the strength development program; that is, as strength improves to the point at which the new weight can be curled more than 15 times without fatigue, it is again replaced with a heavier weight, or with increased resistance if using elastic bands or resistance machines.

The recommended strength training protocol for older adults is that of performing at least one (preferably two) set of 10 to 15 repetitions, to the point of fatigue, for each of the major muscle groups. Important muscle groups for older adults are those needed for lower-body functioning (hip extensors, hip abductors and adductors, knee extensors, and ankle plantar and dorsiflexors), for upper-body functioning (biceps, triceps, shoulders, and back extensors), and for trunk stability (abdominals). Strengthening exercises should be performed at least twice a week with at least 48 hours between sessions. Figures 5.5 and 5.6 provide examples of various types of resistance exercises using body weight, exercise machines, Velcro weights, elastic bands, and hand weights that can be used to improve lower- and upper-body strength in older adults. Additional exercises and information about exercise training for older adults can be found in the resources listed in appendix N.

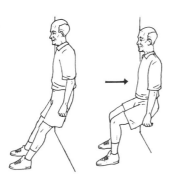

a) Wall Squat. Stand with your back against the wall and your feet about 2 feet (61 cm) away from the wall, and 6 to 8 inches (15 to 20 cm) apart. Slowly slide your back down the wall while bending your knees as illustrated. Hold the position for 10 seconds while continuing to breathe normally, then return to the starting position. Gradually work up to hold the squat for 30 seconds or more.

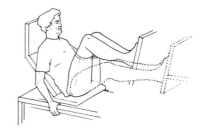

b) Leg Press. From a sitting position with the knees flexed at about 90 degrees and both feet flat on the footrest, extend your legs to the count of 2, pause, and then return slowly to the starting position to the count of 4. The movement should be smooth, not jerky. Be sure to exhale when you push and inhale as you bend your knees. Set the resistance so that you can complete 10 to 15 repetitions.

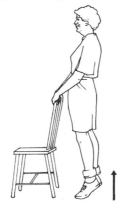

c) Leg Curl. Stand directly behind a chair with your feet flat on the floor, hip-distance apart. Slowly curl your left lower leg up toward your buttocks as illustrated, pause, then return your leg to the starting position. Select a Velcro weight so you can complete 10 to 15 repetitions. When finished, repeat the exercise with your right leg.

d) Leg Extension. Sit squarely and slightly forward on a chair with your feet flat on the floor, hip-distance apart. Slowly extend your lower right leg up to hip level, pause, then slowly return your leg to the starting position. Select a Velcro weight so you can complete 10 to 15 repetitions. When finished, repeat the exercise with your left leg.

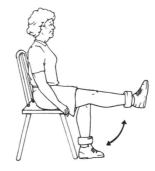

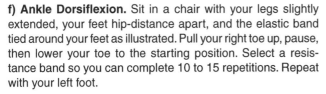

e) Heel Raise. Stand behind a chair with your feet flat on the floor, hip-distance apart. Lift your heels as illustrated, pause, then lower your heels to the starting position. Repeat the exercise between 10 and 15 times. Start off with about 5 lbs (2.3 kg), then gradually add more weight.

f) Ankle Dorsiflexion. Sit in a chair with your legs slightly extended, your feet hip-distance apart, and the elastic band tied around your feet as illustrated. Pull your right toe up, pause, then lower your toe to the starting position. Select a resistance band so you can complete 10 to 15 repetitions. Repeat with your left foot.

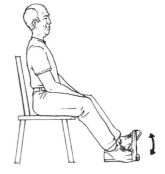

Figure 5.5 Examples of strengthening exercises for the lower body.

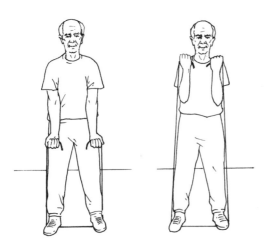

a) Bicep Curl. Standing erect, feet shoulder-width apart and on top of the middle portion of an elastic band or tubing, grasp the tubing with your palms facing forward as illustrated. Slowly bend your arms at the elbows lifting only your forearms up to your shoulders, then slowly return to the starting position. The upper arm should not move. Select a resistance band so you can complete between 10 and 15 repetitions to fatigue.

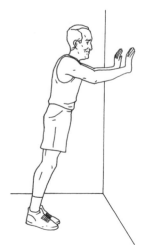

b) Wall Push-Up. Extend your arms and place your hands against the wall, shoulder-width apart. With your arms fully extended, slowly bend your elbows lowering your body toward the wall. Slowly return your arms to the fully extended position without locking your elbows. Repeat the exercise 10 to 15 times. If it is too easy, perform the modified push-up.

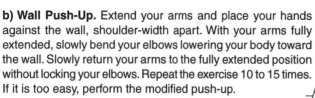

c) Knee Push-Up. Lie on the floor face down with your hands and knees both positioned shoulder-distance apart. Keep back straight and fully extend arms, then bend your elbows lowering your body back to the floor. Complete 10 to 15 repetitions.

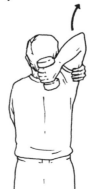

d) Tricep Extension. Position your right arm over your head with your elbow bent and pointed toward the ceiling supported by your other hand as illustrated. Slowly extend your arm toward the ceiling, pause, then slowly return to the starting position. Select a hand weight so you can complete 10 to 15 repetitions to fatigue. Repeat with your left arm.

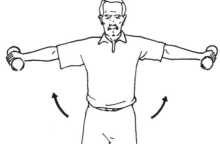

e) Lateral Raise. While holding the weights at your side, slowly lift your arms up to shoulder height as illustrated, pause, then slowly return your arms to the starting position. Select a hand weight that allows you to complete 10 to 15 repetitions to fatigue.

f) Abdominal Crunch. Lie on your back with your head, shoulders, spine, and pelvis gently resting on the floor. Bend your knees, put your feet flat on the floor, and cross your arms over your chest as illustrated. Slowly lift your head, shoulders, and upper torso off the ground, pause, then slowly return to the starting position. Complete as many as you can until fatigue, or until you cannot use correct form.

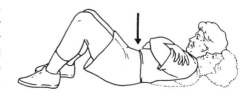

Figure 5.6 Examples of strengthening exercises for the upper body.

Strength Training Guidelines

- Include resistance exercises for each of the major muscle groups.
- Choose a weight (or resistance level) that allows you to perform between 10 and 15 repetitions before fatiguing.
- When you can complete more than 15 reps, increase the amount of weight or resistance.
- Perform at least one set of 10 to 15 reps for each muscle group.
- Perform strength training exercises at least twice a week.

Flexibility. Flexibility is important for maintaining good posture and reducing the risk of injuries and back problems. It is also critical for tasks of daily living such as tying shoes, kneeling down to pick up objects from the floor, putting on overhead garments, and combing hair. In the SFT, lower- and upper-body flexibility is measured using the chair sit-and-reach and the back scratch test items. A well-rounded exercise program should include flexibility exercises for all muscle/joint areas—ankle, knee, hip, back, shoulder, trunk, and neck. We recommend that older adults incorporate stretching into their other daily exercise routines. Before participating in aerobic or strengthening exercise, it is important to first warm up the muscles and joints through walking or light calisthenics and then to do some flexibility exercises to help avoid injuries to the body tissue. Stretching also should be included as part of the cool-down period after exercise sessions.

Stretching exercises should always be performed in a slow and gradual manner, stretching only to the point of mild tension, but not pain. Each stretch should be held at least 5 to 10 seconds and should be repeated at least two or three times. Stretching should never involve bouncing or jerky movements and should never extend beyond the pain-free range of movement. Examples of stretching exercises that are especially suitable as part of the warm-up prior to participating in the SFT are included in figure 4.2. Additional information on flexibility and examples of flexibility exercises can be found in the recommended resources in appendix N.

Flexibility/Stretching Guidelines

- Stretching should be slow and gradual, with no bouncing or jerking.
- Hold each stretch at least 5 to 10 seconds and repeat two or three times.
- Stretching should cause mild tension, but not pain.
- Flexibility exercises should be performed for all major muscle/joint groups: neck, shoulders, back, trunk, hips, knees, ankles.
- Stretching should be included as part of daily exercise routines, and should always occur after muscles are warmed up.

Balance and Agility. Balance and agility are important for a number of common mobility tasks, such as walking; negotiating curbs; climbing stairs; and for making the quick movements needed to avoid hazards in the environment, to get on and off a bus in a timely manner, to cross the street before the light turns red, or to answer a phone or the door. In the SFT, dynamic balance and agility are measured using the 8-foot up-and-go test. Improving balance and agility requires a multidimensional approach that targets the multiple systems contributing to postural control and speed (e.g., sensory, motor, and cognitive). Findings from several studies have shown that balance is best improved, and the risk of falling reduced, if older adults include specific balance and coordination activities in their exercise programs along with aerobic, strength, and flexibility exercises (Province et al., 1995; Rose et al., 1999; Verfaillie et al., 1997).

The best type of exercises to improve balance and agility are those that require the performance of a variety of motor tasks under varying types of sensory and cognitive environments. Examples of such activities, which can range from simple to complex, include standing on one foot with eyes open and with eyes closed, tandem (heel-to-toe) walking, walking on unstable surfaces such as foam pads or rocker boards, and other more complex activities that include quick weight transfers and motor coordination (such as in doing the "grapevine" dance routine). For the more capable older adults, participation in complex exercise-to-music routines and in various sport activities that involve balance and coordination (e.g. tennis or badminton) are excellent ways to maintain balance and agility.

Balance/Agility Training Guidelines

- To improve balance and reduce fall risk, balance/agility activities should be included as part of normal exercise routines.
- Balance/agility is best improved through exercises that involve multiple systems—e.g., sensory, motor, and cognitive.
- Examples of activities that challenge multiple systems include balancing on one foot with eyes open and closed, tandem (heel-to-toe) walking, walking on unstable surfaces (foam pads or rocker boards), and complex aerobic dance and sport activities that involve coordination and balance.

In this section of the chapter we provided suggestions for ways of helping your clients improve their functional fitness and their scores on the SFT. Additional information on exercise programs for older adults can be found in the resources listed in appendix N.

SUMMARY

The performance tables and charts specifically developed for the SFT can assist professionals in the interpretation of test scores. Data from a nationwide study of 7,000 independent-living older adults provide the basis for both norm-referenced and criterion-referenced performance standards as follows:

1. Percentile norm tables provide five-year age group percentile ranks for women and men separately on each of the test items, allowing individuals to compare their scores with those of others of their same age and gender (see appendix H).

2. A "normal range of scores" table provides a simple version of the normative performance scores, giving only the normal ranges of scores (middle 50%) for women and men on each test item (see tables 5.3 and 5.4).

3. SFT performance charts provide a graphic display of data showing the at-risk scoring zones associated with loss of functional mobility for women and men separately on each test item (see figures 5.2 and 5.3).

In interpreting test scores, test users are reminded that the performance standards are based on a select group of volunteer, independent-living older adults throughout the United States who tend to be healthier and more active than the population at large of people over the age of 60.

Administering the SFT can be an effective way of motivating clients to increase their activity participation. For many, just the process of being evaluated is motivating and can cause positive changes in behavior. Test results also can be used as the basis for individual goal-setting and program planning. For some, motivation can be further enhanced by keeping an activity log tracking both program adherence and physical progress. Finally, reevaluation (readministering the SFT at regular intervals) is important in maintaining clients' motivation and interest in their level of physical activity and fitness.

In recommending specific exercises to help clients improve their performance, the following points should be considered:

- Clients' current fitness level and exercise needs (based on SFT scores)
- Clients' personal exercise objectives
- Clients' personal exercise/physical activity preferences (e.g., exercising alone versus in groups, or exercising at home versus in a class or at a fitness center)
- Clients' environmental constraints (e.g., access to facilities, programs, and transportation)
- Data-based exercise recommendations for older adults such as those described in the U.S. surgeon general's report and in the ACSM Position Stand on Exercise and Physical Activity for Older Adults

Recognizing that the best type of exercise is the one that people will do, it is important that clients understand that they can increase their activity level and their fitness in two ways: (1) by increasing the amount of physical activity they get in their normal daily routines, and (2) by participating in a structured exercise program. Although both types of exercise have their advantages and should be encouraged, structured exercise protocols may be needed to address specific weaknesses identified by the SFT scores, particularly for improving aerobic endurance, muscular strength, flexibility, and balance and agility. Because a thorough discussion of exercise programming is beyond the scope of this book, additional resources for helping plan older adult exercise programs are recommended in appendix N.

Informed Consent/Assumption of Liability Form

You are being invited to participate in testing to evaluate your physical fitness. Your participation is entirely voluntary. If you agree to participate, you will be asked to perform a series of assessments designed to evaluate your upper- and lower-body strength, aerobic endurance, flexibility, agility, and balance. These assessments involve activities such as walking, standing, lifting, stepping, and stretching. The risk of engaging in these activities is similar to the risk of engaging in all moderate exercise and may possibly result in muscular fatigue and soreness, sprains and soft tissue injury, skeletal injury, dizziness, and fainting. There is also the risk of cardiac arrest, stroke, and even death.

If any of the following apply, you should not participate in testing without written permission of your physician:

1. Your doctor has advised you not to exercise because of your medical condition(s).

2. You have experienced congestive heart failure.

3. You are currently experiencing joint pain, chest pain, dizziness, or have exertional angina (chest tightness, pressure, pain, heaviness) during exercise.

4. You have uncontrolled high blood pressure (160/100 or above).

During the assessment you will be asked to perform within your physical "comfort zone" and never to push to a point of overexertion or beyond what you feel is safe. You will be instructed to notify the person monitoring your assessment if you feel any discomfort or experience any unusual physical symptoms such as unusual shortness of breath, dizziness, tightness or pain in the chest, irregular heartbeats, numbness, loss of balance, nausea, or blurred vision. If you are accidentally injured during testing, the test administrators will be unable to provide treatment for you other than basic first aid. You will be required to seek treatment from your own physician, which must be paid for by you or your insurance company.

You may discontinue participation in testing whenever you wish by asking to do so. By signing this form, you acknowledge the following:

1. I have read the full content of this document. I have been informed of the purpose of the testing and of the physical risks that I may encounter.

2. I agree to monitor my own physical condition during testing and agree to stop my participation and inform the person administering the assessment if I feel uncomfortable or experience any unusual symptoms.

3. I assume full responsibility for all risk of bodily injury and death as a result of participating in testing. Should I suffer an injury or become ill during testing, I understand that I must seek treatment from my own physician and that I or my insurance company will have to pay for this treatment.

My signature below indicates that I have had an opportunity to ask and have answered any questions I may have, and that I freely consent to participate in the physical assessment.

Signature _____   Date _____

Print Name _____

Medical Clearance Form

Your patient is interested in taking a test battery designed to assess the underlying physical parameters associated with functional mobility (strength, endurance, flexibility, balance, and agility). The test battery was developed and scientifically validated through research at the Ruby Gerontology Center at California State University, Fullerton.

All test items will be administered by trained personnel, and procedures for any medical emergency are in place. Participants will be instructed to do the best they can within their "comfort zone" and never to push themselves to the point of overexertion, or beyond what they think is safe for them. Technicians have been instructed to discontinue testing if at any time participants show signs of dizziness, pain, nausea, or undue fatigue. The test items are:

1. Chair Stand Test (number of stands from a chair in 30 sec)
2. Arm Curl Test (number of curls in 30 sec; 5-lb weight for women, 8-lb weight for men)
3. 6-Minute Walk Test (number of yds walked in 6 min—person can rest when necessary)
4. 2-Minute Step Test (number of steps completed in 2 min)
5. Chair Sit-and-Reach Test (distance one can reach forward toward toes)
6. Back Scratch Test (how far hands can reach behind the back)
7. 8-Foot Up-and-Go Test (time required to get up from a chair, walk 8 ft, and return to chair.

If you know of any medical or other reasons why participation in the fitness testing by your patient would be unwise, please indicate so on this form. By completing the following form, you are not assuming any responsibility for the administration of the test battery.

If you have any questions about the fitness testing, please call _____

____ I know of no reason why my patient should not participate.

____ I believe my patient can participate, but I urge caution because _____

_____

_____

____ My patient should not engage in the following test items:_____

_____

_____

____ I recommend that my patient NOT participate in testing.

Physician Signature _____ Date _____

Print Name of Physician _____ Phone _____

Participant Instructions Prior to Assessment

Place _____

Date _____

Time _____

Although the physical risks associated with the testing are minimal, the following reminders are important in assuring your safety and helping you score the best you can.

1. Avoid strenuous physical activity one or two days prior to assessment.
2. Avoid excess alcohol use for 24 hours prior to testing.
3. Eat a light meal one hour prior to testing.
4. Wear clothing and shoes appropriate for participating in physical activity.
5. Bring a hat and sunglasses for walking outside, and reading glasses (if needed) for completing forms.
6. Bring the Informed Consent/Assumption of Liability and Medical Clearance forms, if required.
7. Inform test administrator of any medical conditions or medications that could affect your performance.

Note: As part of your testing, you will be asked to perform the aerobic endurance test checked below:

____ 6-minute walk test around a flat course to determine the amount of distance you can cover in that time, OR

____ 2-minute step test to see how many times you can step (march) in place in 2 minutes.

After you have determined that it is safe for you to participate in the tests (see Informed Consent/Assumption of Liability form), you should practice the aerobic test checked above at least once before test day—that is, time yourself either walking for 6 minutes or stepping (marching) in place for 2 minutes. This will help you determine the pace that will work best for you on test day.

Scorecard: Senior Fitness Test

Date _____

Name _____ M___ F___ Age _____ Ht _____ Wt _____

Test Item	Trial 1	Trial 2	Comments
1. Chair Stand Test (# in 30 sec)	_____	N/A	
2. Arm Curl Test (# in 30 sec)	_____	N/A	
3. 2-Minute Step Test* (# of steps)	_____	N/A	
4. Chair Sit-and-Reach Test (nearest 1/2 in.: +/-)	_____	_____	Extended leg: R or L
5. Back Scratch Test (nearest 1/2 in.: +/-)	_____	_____	Hand over: R or L shoulder
6. 8-Foot Up-and-Go Test (nearest 1/10 sec)	_____	_____	
6- Minute Walk Test (# of yd)	_____	N/A	

* Omit 2-minute step test if 6-minute walk test is given.

Scorecard: Senior Fitness Test

Date _____

Name _____ M___ F___ Age _____ Ht _____ Wt _____

Test Item	Trial 1	Trial 2	Comments
1. Chair Stand Test (# in 30 sec)	_____	N/A	
2. Arm Curl Test (# in 30 sec)	_____	N/A	
3. 2-Minute Step Test* (# of steps)	_____	N/A	
4. Chair Sit-and-Reach Test (nearest 1/2 in.: +/-)	_____	_____	Extended leg: R or L
5. Back Scratch Test (nearest 1/2 in.: +/-)	_____	_____	Hand over: R or L shoulder
6. 8-Foot Up-and-Go Test (nearest 1/10 sec)	_____	_____	
6- Minute Walk Test (# of yd)	_____	N/A	

* Omit 2-minute step test if 6-minute walk test is given.

Accident Report Form

Date of Injury _____ Time _____ a.m.   p.m.
Date/Month/Year   Hour/Min

Name of Injured Person _____

Address _____

City _____ State _____ Zip Code _____

Gender _____ Age _____ Area Code & Phone # _____

Check suspected cause of injury or illness: ___ Fall   ___ Overexposure

___ Hyperflexion   Other (specify) _____

___ Blunt trauma   ___ Overexertion   ___ Hyperextension

Describe the nature of injury/illness in detail. (Did it happen before, during, or after activity?

How?): _____

_____

Check site of injury/illness: ___ None   ___ Chest/ribs   ___ Hand   ___ Neck/throat
___ Wrist   ___ Abdomen   ___ Ear   ___ Head   ___ Nose   ___ Ankle   ___ Elbow
___ Shoulder/collarbone   ___ Arm   ___ Face   ___ Knee   ___ Stomach
___ Back (upper)   ___ Fingers/thumb   ___ Leg   ___ Teeth   ___ Back (lower)
___ Foot   ___ Mouth   ___ Toes   ___ Other (specify) _____

Check sign and/or symptom: ___ Abrasion   ___ Discoloration   ___ Loss of function
___ Pain   ___ Visual involvement   ___ Contusion   ___ Fracture   ___ Lung involvement
___ Shock   ___ Cut   ___ Heart involvement   ___ Nausea/vomiting   ___ Sprain/strain
___ Dislocation   ___ Internal injury   ___ Numbness   ___ Swelling
___ Other (specify _____

What was done for the injured? _____

_____

By whom? _____

Was the injured person sent to the hospital?   ___ Yes   ___ No

Was the injured person sent to a physician?   ___ Yes   ___ No

To whom was injured person released   ___ Self   ___ Relative   ___ Other (specify) ___

_____

Signature of Person Filling Out Form _____ Date _____

Witness Signature _____ Date _____

APPENDIX F
BMI Conversion Chart

Weight (lb)	Height (in.)																	
	49	51	53	55	57	59	61	63	65	67	69	71	73	75	77	79	81	83
66	19	18	16	15	14	13	12	12	11	10	10	9	9	8	8	8	7	7
70	20	19	18	16	15	14	13	13	12	11	10	10	9	9	8	8	8	7
75	22	20	19	17	16	15	14	13	12	12	11	10	10	9	9	9	8	8
79	23	21	20	18	17	16	15	14	13	12	12	11	11	10	9	9	9	8
84	24	22	21	19	18	17	16	15	14	13	12	12	11	11	10	10	9	9
88	26	24	22	20	19	18	17	16	15	14	13	12	12	11	11	10	10	9
92	27	25	23	21	20	19	17	16	15	15	14	13	12	12	11	11	10	10
97	28	26	24	22	21	20	18	17	16	15	14	14	13	12	12	11	10	10
101	29	27	25	23	22	20	19	18	17	16	15	14	13	13	12	12	11	10
106	31	28	26	24	23	21	20	19	18	17	16	15	14	13	13	12	11	11
110	32	30	27	26	24	22	21	20	18	17	16	15	15	14	13	13	11	11
114	33	31	29	27	25	23	22	20	19	18	17	16	15	14	14	13	12	12
119	35	32	30	28	26	24	22	21	20	19	18	17	16	15	14	14	13	12
123	36	33	31	29	27	25	23	22	21	19	18	17	16	16	15	14	13	13
128	37	34	32	30	28	26	24	23	21	20	19	18	17	16	15	15	14	13
132	38	36	33	31	29	27	25	23	22	21	20	19	18	17	16	15	14	14
136	40	37	34	32	29	28	26	24	23	21	20	19	18	17	16	16	15	14
141	41	38	35	33	30	28	27	25	24	22	21	20	19	18	17	16	15	15
145	42	39	36	34	31	29	27	26	24	23	22	20	19	18	17	17	16	15
150	44	40	37	35	32	30	28	27	25	24	22	21	20	19	18	17	16	15
154	45	41	38	36	33	31	29	27	26	24	23	22	20	19	18	18	17	16
158	46	43	40	37	34	32	30	28	26	25	24	22	21	20	19	18	17	16
163	47	44	41	38	35	33	31	29	27	26	24	23	22	20	19	19	18	17
167	49	45	42	39	36	34	32	30	28	26	25	23	22	21	20	19	18	17
172	50	46	43	40	37	35	32	30	29	27	25	24	23	22	21	20	19	18
176	51	47	44	41	38	36	33	31	29	28	26	25	23	22	21	20	19	18
180	52	49	45	42	39	36	34	32	30	28	27	25	24	23	22	21	20	19
185	54	50	46	43	40	37	35	33	31	29	27	26	25	23	22	21	20	19
189	55	51	47	44	41	38	36	34	32	30	28	27	25	24	23	22	20	20
194	56	52	48	45	42	39	37	34	32	30	29	27	26	24	23	22	21	20
198	58	53	49	46	43	40	37	35	33	31	29	28	26	25	24	23	21	20
202	59	54	50	47	44	41	38	36	34	32	30	28	27	25	24	23	22	21
207	60	56	52	48	45	42	39	37	35	33	31	29	27	26	25	24	22	21
211	61	57	53	49	46	43	40	38	35	33	31	30	28	27	25	24	23	22
216	63	58	54	50	47	44	41	38	36	34	32	30	29	27	26	25	23	22
220	64	59	55	51	48	44	42	39	37	35	33	31	29	28	26	25	24	23
224	65	60	56	52	49	45	42	40	37	35	33	31	30	28	27	26	24	23
229	67	62	57	53	49	46	43	41	38	36	34	32	30	29	27	26	25	24
233	68	63	58	54	50	47	44	41	39	37	35	33	31	29	28	27	25	24
238	69	64	59	55	51	48	45	42	40	37	35	33	32	30	28	27	26	24
242	70	65	60	56	52	49	46	43	40	38	36	34	32	30	29	28	26	25
246	72	66	61	57	53	50	47	44	41	39	37	35	33	31	29	28	27	25
251	73	67	63	58	54	51	47	45	42	39	37	35	33	32	30	29	27	26
255	74	69	64	59	55	52	48	45	43	40	38	36	34	32	31	29	28	26
260	76	70	65	60	56	52	49	46	43	41	39	36	34	33	31	30	28	27
264	77	71	66	61	57	53	50	47	44	42	39	37	35	33	32	30	29	27
268	78	72	67	62	58	54	51	48	45	42	40	38	36	34	32	31	29	28
273	79	73	68	63	59	55	52	48	46	43	40	38	36	34	33	31	30	28
277	81	75	69	64	60	56	52	49	46	44	41	39	37	35	33	32	30	29
282	82	76	70	65	61	57	53	50	47	44	42	40	37	35	34	32	30	29

Body mass index (BMI) is determined by locating the point at which the horizontal row indicating a person's weight intersects with the vertical column indicating the person's height. BMI values of 19 to 26 generally are considered to be in the healthy range. Values above or below the shaded area may be associated with increased risk for disease and loss of mobility in later years (American College of Sports Medicine, 1998b; Evans & Rosenberg, 1991; Galanos et al., 1994; Harris et al., 1989; Losonczy et al., 1995; Shephard, 1997).

Appendix G

Station Signs for Posting

1. **Chair Stand Test**

2. **Arm Curl Test**

3a. **Height and Weight**

3b. **2-Minute Step Test**

4. **Chair Sit-and-Reach Test**

5. **Back Scratch Test**

6. **8-Foot Up-and-Go Test**

   6-Minute Walk Test*

* If the 6-minute walk test is used as the test of aerobic endurance, omit the 2-minute step test. Administer the 6-minute walk test after all other tests are completed.

STATION 1

CHAIR STAND TEST

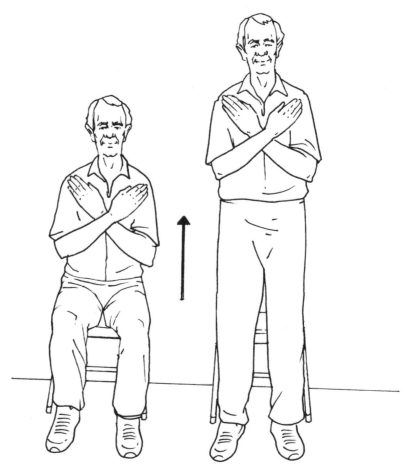

PURPOSE:

To measure lower-body strength

EQUIPMENT:

Straight-back chair (17 in. or 43.18 cm seat height); stopwatch

PROCEDURE:

- Have the participant sit in the middle of the chair, feet flat on the floor, arms across chest.
- On signal "go" have the participant rise to a full stand, then return to a fully seated position.
- After a warm-up trial to check for correct form, administer one test trial.
- The score is the number of stands completed in 30 seconds.

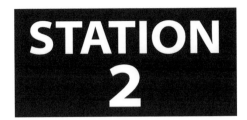

ARM CURL TEST

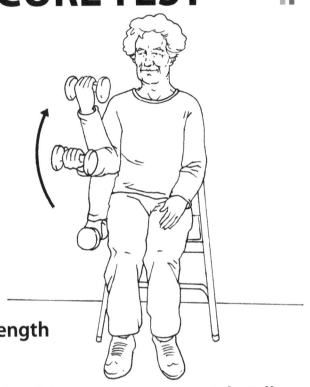

PURPOSE:

To measure upper-body strength

EQUIPMENT:

Straight-back or folding chair without arms, stopwatch, 5-lb and 8-lb dumbbells

PROCEDURE:

- Have the participant sit in the chair (slightly to the dominant side), with feet flat on the floor.

- The participant should hold the weight down at the side, perpendicular to the floor, in a handshake grip.

- On the signal "go" have the participant curl the weight through a full range of motion as many times as possible in 30 seconds. The palm should rotate up during the curl-up phase, then should return to a handshake position at extension. The upper arm must remain still throughout the test.

- After one or two warm-up curls without the weight to check for correct form, administer one test trial.

- The score is the number of curls completed in 30 seconds.

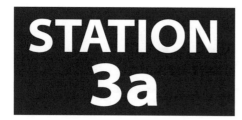

STATION 3a

HEIGHT AND WEIGHT

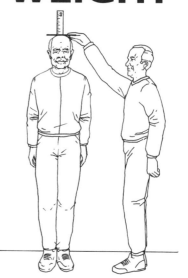

PURPOSE:

To assess body mass index (BMI)

EQUIPMENT:

Scale, 60-in (152.4-cm) tape measure, masking tape, and ruler (or other flat object to mark top of head)

PROCEDURE: (weight)

- Have the participant remove any heavy coats or sweaters; shoes may be left on.

- Measure weight to the nearest pound, subtracting 1 to 2 lbs (1/2 to 1 kg) for shoes.

PROCEDURE: (height)

- Position the tape measure on the wall, 20 in. (50.8 cm) up from the floor.

- Have the participant stand against the wall with the back of the head lined up with the tape measure.

- Lay the ruler on top of the participant's head, extending it back to the tape measure.

- The score is the number of inches in height as indicated on the tape measure, plus 20 in. (50.8 cm) (the distance from the floor to the zero mark on the tape).

- If shoes were worn, subtract 1 to 2 in. (2 to 4 cm), using your best judgment.

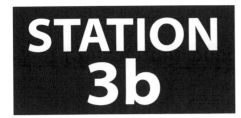

2-MINUTE STEP TEST

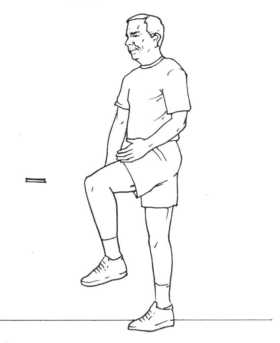

PURPOSE:

To assess aerobic endurance

EQUIPMENT:

Tally counter, stopwatch, tape measure or 30-in. (76.2-cm) piece of cord, masking tape

PROCEDURE:

- To establish stepping height, use masking tape to mark the midpoint between the participant's kneecap and iliac crest (front protruding hip bone), which you can determine by extending the cord between the middle of the patella and the hip bone, then doubling it over.

- Transfer the masking tape to a nearby wall or doorway to use as a guide for the correct stepping height.

- On the signal "go" the participant should begin stepping in place, raising each knee to the indicated height.

- The score is the number of full steps completed in 2 minutes (counted each time the right knee reaches the target height).

STATION 4

CHAIR SIT-AND-REACH TEST

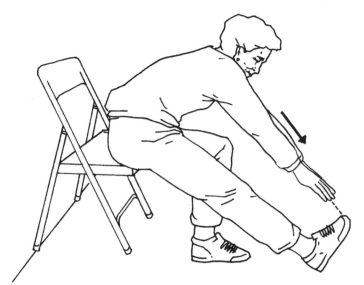

PURPOSE:

To assess lower-body (primarily hamstring) flexibility

EQUIPMENT:

Folding chair with a seat height of 17 in. (43.18 cm) that will not tip forward, 18-in. (45.72-cm) ruler (half a yardstick).

PROCEDURE:

- Have the participant sit on the edge of the chair, with the crease at the top of the leg even with the chair.

- The preferred leg should be extended straight out in front of the hip, with the heel on the floor and the ankle flexed at 90°; the other leg is bent and off to the side, with the foot flat on the floor. (The preferred leg is the one resulting in the better score.)

- With hands overlapping and the middle fingers even, have the participant reach toward the toes as far as possible.

- After two practice trials, administer two test trials and record scores to the nearest half inch. Record a minus (–) score if the reach is short of the toes and a plus (+) score if the reach goes beyond the toes.

- The knee of the extended leg *must* remain straight.

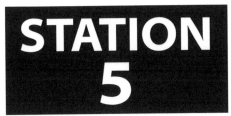

BACK SCRATCH TEST

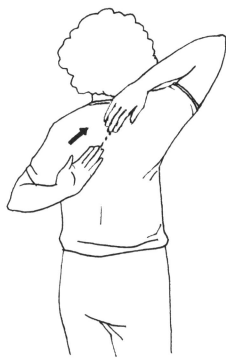

PURPOSE:
To measure upper-body flexibility

EQUIPMENT:
18-in. (45.72-cm) ruler (half a yardstick)

PROCEDURE:
- Have the participant reach one hand over the shoulder and down the back; the other around the back and up the middle.
- Have the participant practice to determine the preferred position (best hand over the top).
- After two warm-up practice trials, administer two test trials, measuring the distance between the middle fingers.
- Record scores to the nearest half inch (1 cm). Minus scores (–) represent the distance short of touching the middle fingers; plus scores (+) indicate the degree of overlap. Circle the better score.

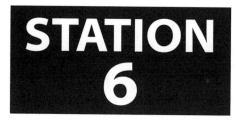

8-FOOT UP-AND-GO TEST

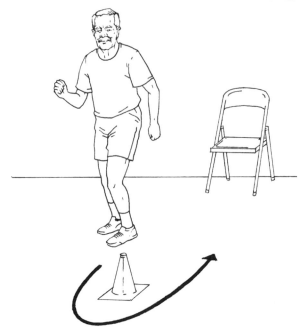

PURPOSE:

To assess agility and dynamic balance

EQUIPMENT:

Folding chair with 17-in. (43.18-cm) seat height, stopwatch, tape measure, and cone (or similar marker)

PROCEDURE:

- Have the participant sit in the middle of the chair, hands on thighs, one foot slightly ahead of the other, body leaning slightly forward.

- On the signal "go" have the participant get up from the chair, walk as quickly as possible around a cone placed 8 feet away, and return to the chair.

- The timer must start the stopwatch exactly on the "go" signal and stop it at the exact time the participant sits in the chair.

- After one practice trial, administer two test trials. The score is the best of two trials, recorded to the nearest tenth of a second.

6-MINUTE WALK TEST

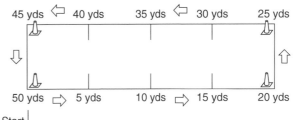

45 yds ⇐ 40 yds   35 yds ⇐ 30 yds   25 yds

⇩   ⇧

50 yds ⇨ 5 yds   10 yds ⇨ 15 yds   20 yds

PURPOSE:

To assess aerobic endurance

Start |

EQUIPMENT:

Long measuring tape, two stopwatches, four cones, masking tape, popsicle sticks or index cards and pencils (to count laps walked), chairs for waiting participants, name tags

SETUP:

Mark off 50-yard course (20 yards by 5 yards) into 5-yard segments. In metric units, the course is 45.7 meters marked off by 4.57-meter segments.

PROCEDURE:

- Partner-up all participants, using name tags to indicate partner number.

- One partner in each group lines up at the start line for testing. Waiting partners count laps, either by handing the walker a popsicle stick each time a lap is completed or by marking laps on a card.

- Starting (and stopping) times are staggered 10 seconds apart. On signal "go" walkers start one at a time, then walk as fast as they can (within their comfort zone) trying to cover as many yards (laps) as possible in 6 minutes.

- At the end of 6 minutes, stop walkers (one at a time) and have them move to the side. The score is the number of laps walked multiplied by 50 yards (or 45.7 meters), plus the number of extra yards or meters (indicated by the closest 5-yard or 4.57-meter marker).

Appendix H

Age Group Percentile Norms

Chair Stand Test

Arm Curl Test

6-Minute Walk Test

2-Minute Step Test

Chair Sit-and-Reach Test

Back Scratch Test

8-Foot Up-and-Go Test

Chair Stand Test (Women)

Percentile rank	60–64	65–69	70–74	75–79	80–84	85–89	90–94
95	21	19	19	19	18	17	16
90	20	18	18	17	17	15	15
85	19	17	17	16	16	14	13
80	18	16	16	16	15	14	12
75	17	16	15	15	14	13	11
70	17	15	15	14	13	12	11
65	16	15	14	14	13	12	10
60	16	14	14	13	12	11	9
55	15	14	13	13	12	11	9
50	15	14	13	12	11	10	8
45	14	13	12	12	11	10	7
40	14	13	12	12	10	9	7
35	13	12	11	11	10	9	6
30	12	12	11	11	9	8	5
25	12	11	10	10	9	8	4
20	11	11	10	9	8	7	4
15	10	10	9	9	7	6	3
10	9	9	8	8	6	5	1
5	8	8	7	6	4	4	0

Adapted from Rikli & Jones 1999.

Chair Stand Test (Men)

Percentile rank	60–64	65–69	70–74	75–79	80–84	85–89	90–94
95	23	23	21	21	19	19	16
90	22	21	20	20	17	17	15
85	21	20	19	18	16	16	14
80	20	19	18	18	16	15	13
75	19	18	17	17	15	14	12
70	19	18	17	16	14	13	12
65	18	17	16	16	14	13	11
60	17	16	16	15	13	12	11
55	17	16	15	15	13	12	10
50	16	15	14	14	12	11	10
45	16	15	14	13	12	11	9
40	15	14	13	13	11	10	9
35	15	13	13	12	11	9	8
30	14	13	12	12	10	9	8
25	14	12	12	11	10	8	7
20	13	11	11	10	9	7	7
15	12	11	10	10	8	6	6
10	11	9	9	8	7	5	5
5	9	8	8	7	6	4	3

Adapted from Rikli & Jones 1999.

Arm Curl Test (Women)

Percentile rank	60–64	65–69	70–74	75–79	80–84	85–89	90–94
95	24	22	22	21	20	18	17
90	22	21	20	20	18	17	16
85	21	20	19	19	17	16	15
80	20	19	18	18	16	15	14
75	19	18	17	17	16	15	13
70	18	17	17	16	15	14	13
65	18	17	16	16	15	14	12
60	17	16	16	15	14	13	12
55	17	16	15	15	14	13	11
50	16	15	14	14	13	12	11
45	16	15	14	13	12	12	10
40	15	14	13	13	12	11	10
35	14	14	13	12	11	11	9
30	14	13	12	12	11	10	9
25	13	12	12	11	10	10	8
20	12	12	11	10	10	9	8
15	11	11	10	9	9	8	7
10	10	10	9	8	8	7	6
5	9	8	8	7	6	6	5

Adapted from Rikli & Jones 1999.

Arm Curl Test (Men)

Percentile rank	60–64	65–69	70–74	75–79	80–84	85–89	90–94
95	27	27	26	24	23	21	18
90	25	25	24	22	22	19	16
85	24	24	23	21	20	18	16
80	23	23	22	20	20	17	15
75	22	21	21	19	19	17	14
70	21	21	20	19	18	16	14
65	21	20	19	18	18	15	13
60	20	20	19	17	17	15	13
55	20	19	18	17	17	14	12
50	19	18	17	16	16	14	12
45	18	18	17	16	15	13	12
40	18	17	16	15	15	13	11
35	17	16	15	14	14	12	11
30	17	16	15	14	14	11	10
25	16	15	14	13	13	11	10
20	15	14	13	12	12	10	9
15	14	13	12	11	12	9	8
10	13	12	11	10	10	8	8
5	11	10	9	9	9	7	6

Adapted from Rikli & Jones 1999.

6-Minute Walk Test (Women)

Percentile rank	60–64	65–69	70–74	75–79	80–84	85–89	90–94
95	741	734	709	696	654	638	564
90	711	697	673	655	612	591	518
85	690	673	650	628	584	560	488
80	674	653	630	605	560	534	463
75	659	636	614	585	540	512	441
70	647	621	599	568	523	493	423
65	636	607	586	553	508	476	406
60	624	593	572	538	491	458	388
55	614	581	561	524	477	443	373
50	603	568	548	509	462	426	357
45	592	555	535	494	447	409	341
40	582	543	524	480	433	394	326
35	570	529	510	465	416	376	308
30	559	515	497	450	401	359	291
25	547	500	482	433	384	340	273
20	532	483	466	413	364	318	251
15	516	463	446	390	340	292	226
10	495	439	423	363	312	261	196
5	465	402	387	322	270	214	150

Adapted from Rikli & Jones 1999.

6-Minute Walk Test (Men)

Percentile rank	60–64	65–69	70–74	75–79	80–84	85–89	90–94
95	825	800	779	762	721	710	646
90	792	763	743	716	678	659	592
85	770	738	718	686	649	625	557
80	751	718	698	661	625	596	527
75	736	700	680	639	604	572	502
70	722	685	665	621	586	551	480
65	710	671	652	604	571	532	461
60	697	657	638	586	554	512	440
55	686	644	625	571	540	495	422
50	674	631	612	555	524	477	403
45	662	618	599	539	508	459	384
40	651	605	586	524	494	442	366
35	638	591	572	506	477	422	345
30	626	577	559	489	462	403	326
25	612	562	544	471	444	382	304
20	597	544	526	449	423	358	279
15	578	524	506	424	399	329	249
10	556	499	481	394	370	295	214
5	523	462	445	348	327	244	160

Adapted from Rikli & Jones 1999.

2-Minute Step Test (Women)

Percentile rank	60–64	65–69	70–74	75–79	80–84	85–89	90–94
95	130	133	125	123	113	106	92
90	122	123	116	115	104	98	85
85	116	117	110	109	99	93	80
80	111	112	105	104	94	88	76
75	107	107	101	100	90	85	72
70	103	104	97	96	87	81	69
65	100	100	94	93	84	79	66
60	97	96	90	90	81	76	63
55	94	93	87	87	78	73	61
50	91	90	84	84	75	70	58
45	88	87	81	81	72	67	55
40	85	84	78	78	69	64	53
35	82	80	74	75	66	61	50
30	79	76	71	72	63	59	47
25	75	73	68	68	60	55	44
20	71	68	63	64	56	52	40
15	66	63	58	59	51	47	36
10	60	57	52	53	46	42	31
5	52	47	43	45	37	39	24

Adapted from Rikli & Jones 1999.

2-Minute Step Test (Men)

Percentile rank	60–64	65–69	70–74	75–79	80–84	85–89	90–94
95	135	139	133	135	126	114	112
90	128	130	124	126	118	106	102
85	123	125	119	119	112	100	96
80	119	120	114	114	107	95	91
75	115	116	110	109	103	91	86
70	112	113	107	105	99	87	83
65	109	110	104	102	96	84	79
60	106	107	101	98	93	81	76
55	104	104	98	95	90	78	72
50	101	101	95	91	87	75	69
45	98	98	92	87	84	72	66
40	96	95	89	84	81	69	62
35	93	92	86	80	78	66	59
30	90	89	83	77	75	63	55
25	87	86	80	73	71	59	52
20	83	82	76	68	67	55	47
15	79	77	71	63	62	50	42
10	74	72	66	56	56	44	36
5	67	67	67	47	48	36	26

Adapted from Rikli & Jones 1999.

Chair Sit-and-Reach Test (Women)

Percentile rank	60–64	65–69	70–74	75–79	80–84	85–89	90–94
95	8.7	7.9	7.5	7.4	6.6	6.0	4.9
90	7.2	6.6	6.1	6.1	5.2	4.6	3.4
85	6.3	5.7	5.2	5.2	4.3	3.7	2.5
80	5.5	5.0	4.5	4.4	3.6	3.0	1.7
75	4.8	4.4	3.9	3.7	3.0	2.4	1.0
70	4.2	3.9	3.3	3.2	2.4	1.8	0.4
65	3.7	3.4	2.8	2.7	1.9	1.3	−0.1
60	3.1	2.9	2.3	2.1	1.4	0.8	−0.7
55	2.6	2.5	1.9	1.7	1.0	0.4	−1.2
50	2.1	2.0	1.4	1.2	0.5	−0.1	−1.7
45	1.6	1.5	0.9	0.7	0.0	−0.6	−2.2
40	1.1	1.1	0.5	0.2	−0.4	−1.0	−2.7
35	0.5	0.6	0.0	−0.3	−0.9	−1.5	−3.3
30	0.0	0.1	−0.5	−0.8	−1.4	−2.0	−3.8
25	−0.6	−0.4	−1.1	−1.3	−2.0	−2.6	−4.4
20	−1.3	−1.0	−1.7	−2.0	−2.6	−3.2	−5.1
15	−2.1	−1.7	−2.4	−2.8	−3.3	−3.9	−5.9
10	−3.0	−2.6	−3.3	−3.7	−4.2	−4.8	−6.8
5	−4.0	−3.9	−4.7	−5.0	−5.0	−6.3	−7.9

Adapted from Rikli & Jones 1999.

Chair Sit-and-Reach Test (Men)

Percentile rank	60–64	65–69	70–74	75–79	80–84	85–89	90–94
95	8.5	7.5	7.5	6.6	6.2	4.5	3.5
90	6.7	5.9	5.8	4.9	4.4	3.0	1.9
85	5.6	4.8	4.7	3.8	3.2	2.0	0.9
80	4.6	3.9	3.8	2.8	2.2	1.1	0.0
75	3.8	3.1	3.0	2.0	1.4	0.4	−0.7
70	3.1	2.4	2.4	1.3	0.6	−0.2	−1.4
65	2.5	1.8	1.8	0.7	0.0	−0.8	−1.9
60	1.8	1.1	1.1	0.1	−0.8	−1.3	−2.5
55	1.2	0.6	0.6	−0.5	−1.4	−1.9	−3.0
50	0.6	0.0	0.0	−1.1	−2.0	−2.4	−3.6
45	0.0	−0.6	−0.6	−1.7	−2.6	−2.9	−4.2
40	−0.6	−1.1	−1.2	−2.3	−3.2	−3.5	−4.7
35	−1.3	−1.8	−1.8	−2.9	−4.0	−4.0	−5.3
30	−1.9	−2.4	−2.4	−3.5	−4.6	−4.6	−5.8
25	−2.6	−3.1	−3.1	−4.2	−5.3	−5.3	−6.5
20	−3.4	−3.9	−3.9	−5.0	−6.2	−5.9	−7.2
15	−4.4	−4.8	−4.8	−6.0	−7.2	−6.8	−8.1
10	−5.5	−5.9	−5.9	−7.1	−8.4	−7.8	−9.1
5	−7.3	−7.5	−7.6	−8.8	−10.2	−9.3	−10.7

Adapted from Rikli & Jones 1999.

Back Scratch Test (Women)

Percentile rank	60–64	65–69	70–74	75–79	80–84	85–89	90–94
95	5.0	4.9	4.5	4.5	4.3	3.5	3.9
90	3.8	3.5	3.2	3.1	2.8	1.9	2.2
85	2.9	2.6	2.3	2.2	1.8	0.8	0.9
80	2.2	1.9	1.5	1.3	0.9	−0.1	−0.1
75	1.6	1.3	0.8	0.6	0.2	−0.9	−1.0
70	1.1	0.7	0.3	0.0	−0.4	−1.6	−1.8
65	0.7	0.2	−0.2	−0.5	−1.0	−2.1	−2.5
60	0.2	−0.3	−0.8	−1.1	−1.6	−2.8	−3.2
55	−0.2	−0.7	−1.2	−1.6	−2.1	−3.3	−3.8
50	−0.7	−1.2	−1.7	−2.1	−2.6	−3.9	−4.5
45	−1.2	−1.7	−2.2	−2.6	−3.1	−4.5	−5.2
40	−1.6	−2.1	−2.6	−3.1	−3.7	−5.0	−5.8
35	−2.1	−2.6	−3.2	−3.7	−4.2	−5.7	−6.5
30	−2.5	−3.1	−3.7	−4.2	−4.8	−6.2	−7.2
25	−3.0	−3.7	−4.2	−4.8	−5.4	−6.9	−8.0
20	−3.6	−4.3	−4.9	−5.5	−6.1	−7.7	−8.9
15	−4.3	−5.0	−5.7	−6.4	−7.0	−8.6	−9.9
10	−5.2	−5.9	−6.6	−7.3	−8.0	−9.7	−11.2
5	−6.4	−7.3	−7.9	−8.8	−9.5	−11.3	−13.0

Adapted from Rikli & Jones 1999.

Back Scratch Test (Men)

Percentile rank	60–64	65–69	70–74	75–79	80–84	85–89	90–94
95	4.5	3.9	3.5	2.8	3.2	1.7	0.7
90	2.7	2.2	1.8	0.9	1.2	−0.1	−1.1
85	1.6	1.0	0.6	−0.3	−0.1	−1.2	−2.2
80	0.6	0.0	−0.4	−1.3	−1.2	−2.2	−3.2
75	−0.2	−0.8	−1.2	−2.2	−2.1	−3.0	−4.0
70	−0.9	−1.6	−2.0	−2.9	−2.9	−3.7	−4.7
65	−1.5	−2.2	−2.6	−3.6	−3.6	−4.3	−5.3
60	−2.2	−2.9	−3.3	−4.3	−4.3	−5.0	−6.0
55	−2.8	−3.5	−3.9	−4.9	−5.0	−5.6	−6.6
50	−3.4	−4.1	−4.5	−5.6	−5.7	−6.2	−7.2
45	−4.0	−4.7	−5.1	−6.3	−6.4	−6.8	−7.8
40	−4.6	−5.3	−5.7	−6.9	−7.1	−7.4	−8.4
35	−5.3	−6.0	−6.4	−7.6	−7.8	−8.1	−9.1
30	−5.9	−6.6	−7.0	−8.3	−8.5	−8.7	−9.7
25	−6.6	−7.4	−7.8	−9.0	−9.3	−9.4	−10.4
20	−7.4	−8.2	−8.6	−9.9	−10.2	−10.2	−11.2
15	−8.4	−9.2	−9.6	−10.9	−11.3	−11.2	−12.2
10	−9.5	−10.4	−10.8	−12.1	−12.6	−12.3	−13.3
5	−11.3	−12.1	−12.5	−14.0	−14.6	−14.1	−15.1

Adapted from Rikli & Jones 1999.

8-Foot Up-and-Go Test (Women)

Percentile rank	60–64	65–69	70–74	75–79	80–84	85–89	90–94
95	3.2	3.6	3.8	4.0	4.0	4.5	5.0
90	3.7	4.1	4.0	4.3	4.4	4.7	5.3
85	4.0	4.4	4.3	4.6	4.9	5.3	6.1
80	4.2	4.6	4.7	5.0	5.4	5.8	6.7
75	4.4	4.8	4.9	5.2	5.7	6.2	7.3
70	4.6	5.0	5.2	5.5	6.1	6.6	7.7
65	4.7	5.1	5.4	5.7	6.3	6.9	8.2
60	4.9	5.3	5.6	5.9	6.7	7.3	8.6
55	5.0	5.4	5.8	6.1	6.9	7.6	9.0
50	5.2	5.6	6.0	6.3	7.2	7.9	9.4
45	5.4	5.8	6.2	6.5	7.5	8.2	9.8
40	5.5	5.9	6.4	6.7	7.8	8.5	10.2
35	5.7	6.1	6.6	6.9	8.1	8.9	10.6
30	5.8	6.2	6.8	7.1	8.3	9.2	11.1
25	6.0	6.4	7.1	7.4	8.7	9.6	11.5
20	6.2	6.6	7.3	7.6	9.0	10.0	12.1
15	6.4	6.8	7.7	8.0	9.5	10.5	12.7
10	6.7	7.1	8.0	8.3	10.0	11.1	13.5
5	7.2	7.6	8.6	8.9	10.8	12.0	14.6

Adapted from Rikli & Jones 1999.

8-Foot Up-and-Go Test (Men)

Percentile rank	60–64	65–69	70–74	75–79	80–84	85–89	90–94
95	3.0	3.1	3.2	3.3	4.0	4.0	4.3
90	3.0	3.6	3.6	3.5	4.1	4.3	4.5
85	3.3	3.9	3.9	3.9	4.5	4.5	5.1
80	3.6	4.1	4.2	4.3	4.9	5.0	5.7
75	3.8	4.3	4.4	4.6	5.2	5.5	6.2
70	4.0	4.5	4.6	4.9	5.5	5.8	6.6
65	4.2	4.6	4.8	5.2	5.7	6.2	7.0
60	4.4	4.8	5.0	5.4	6.0	6.5	7.4
55	4.5	4.9	5.1	5.7	6.2	6.9	7.7
50	4.7	5.1	5.3	5.9	6.4	7.2	8.1
45	4.9	5.3	5.5	6.1	6.6	7.5	8.5
40	5.0	5.4	5.6	6.4	6.9	7.9	8.8
35	5.2	5.6	5.8	6.6	7.1	8.2	9.2
30	5.4	5.7	6.0	6.9	7.3	8.6	9.6
25	5.6	5.9	6.2	7.2	7.6	8.9	10.0
20	5.8	6.1	6.4	7.5	7.9	9.4	10.5
15	6.1	6.3	6.7	7.9	8.3	9.9	11.1
10	6.4	6.6	7.0	8.3	8.7	10.5	11.8
5	6.8	7.1	7.4	9.0	9.4	11.5	12.9

Adapted from Rikli & Jones 1999.

Personal Profile Form

Name _____

Age _____ M ____ F ____

Test Date: _____

Test Item	Score	Rating* Below average ◄– – – 25th%	Normal range	Above average 75th% – – – ►	%ile rank[†]	Comments
Chair Stand (No. of stands)			____			
Arm Curl (No. of repetitions)			____			
6-Minute Walk (yd) or **2-Minute Step** (steps)			____			
Chair Sit-&-Reach (No. of in. +/–)			____			
Back Scratch (No. of in. +/–)			____			
8-Foot Up-&-Go (No. of sec)			____			
Body Mass Index (See BMI chart)	Ht ____ Wt ____	BMI ____			≤18 Underweight, may signify loss of muscle or bone 19–26 Healthy range ≥27 Overweight, may cause increased risk of disability/disease	

* Rating categories can be determined from tables 5.3 and 5.4 and are illustrated in the SFT performance charts (see figures 5.2 and 5.3).
† Percentile ranks are determined from tables in appendix H.

Appendix J

Performance Charts

Chair Stand Test

Arm Curl Test

6-Minute Walk Test

2-Minute Step Test

Chair Sit-and-Reach Test

Back Scratch Test

8-Foot Up-and-Go Test

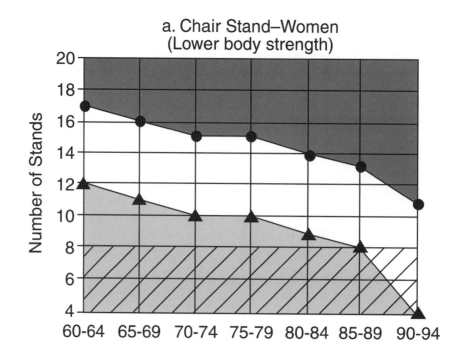

a. Chair Stand–Women
(Lower body strength)

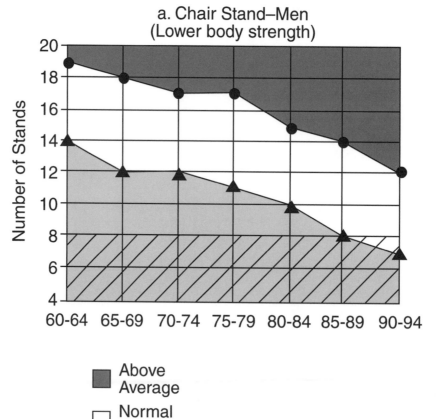

a. Chair Stand–Men
(Lower body strength)

Above Average

Normal Range

Below Average

At risk for loss of functional mobility

● 75th percentile
▲ 25th percentile

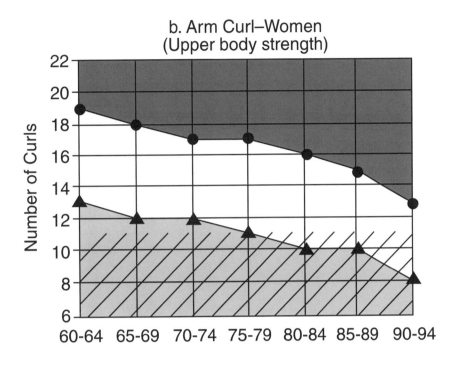

b. Arm Curl–Women
(Upper body strength)

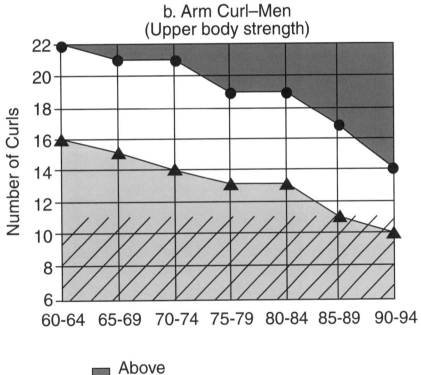

b. Arm Curl–Men
(Upper body strength)

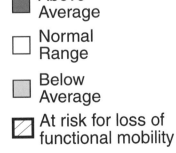

Above Average

Normal Range

Below Average

At risk for loss of functional mobility

75th percentile
25th percentile

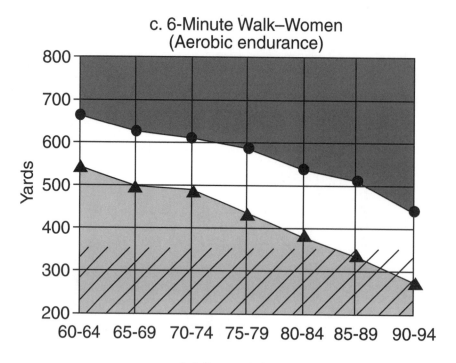

c. 6-Minute Walk–Women
(Aerobic endurance)

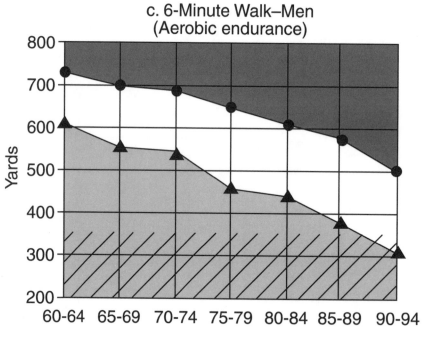

c. 6-Minute Walk–Men
(Aerobic endurance)

Above Average

Normal Range

Below Average

At risk for loss of functional mobility

● 75th percentile
▲ 25th percentile

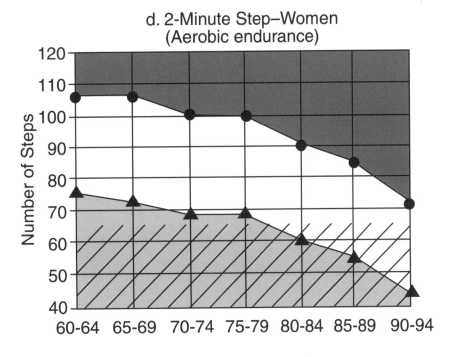

d. 2-Minute Step–Women
(Aerobic endurance)

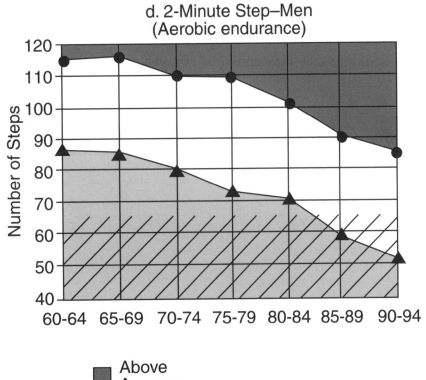

d. 2-Minute Step–Men
(Aerobic endurance)

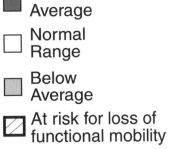

Above Average

Normal Range

Below Average

At risk for loss of functional mobility

● 75th percentile
▲ 25th percentile

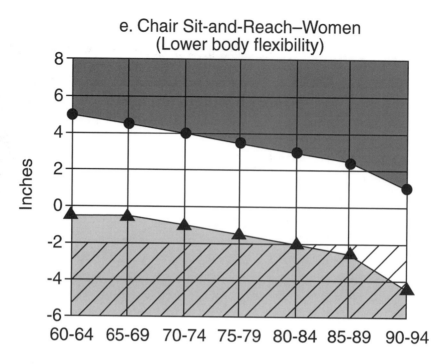

e. Chair Sit-and-Reach–Women
(Lower body flexibility)

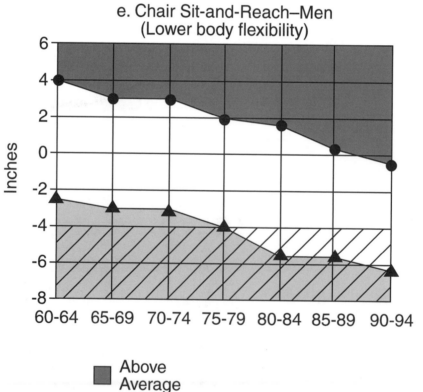

e. Chair Sit-and-Reach–Men
(Lower body flexibility)

Above Average

Normal Range

Below Average

At risk for loss of functional mobility

75th percentile
25th percentile

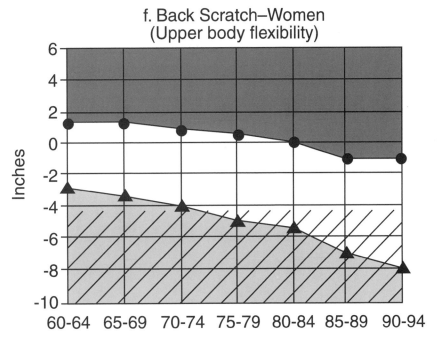

f. Back Scratch–Women
(Upper body flexibility)

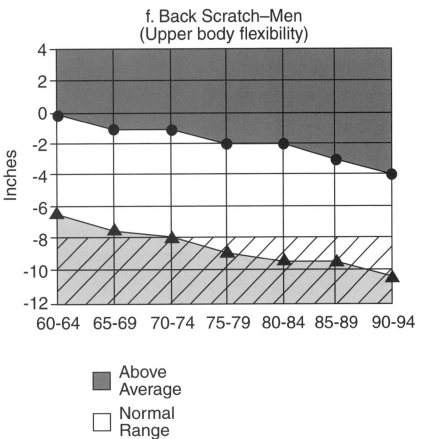

f. Back Scratch–Men
(Upper body flexibility)

Above Average

Normal Range

Below Average

At risk for loss of functional mobility

75th percentile
25th percentile

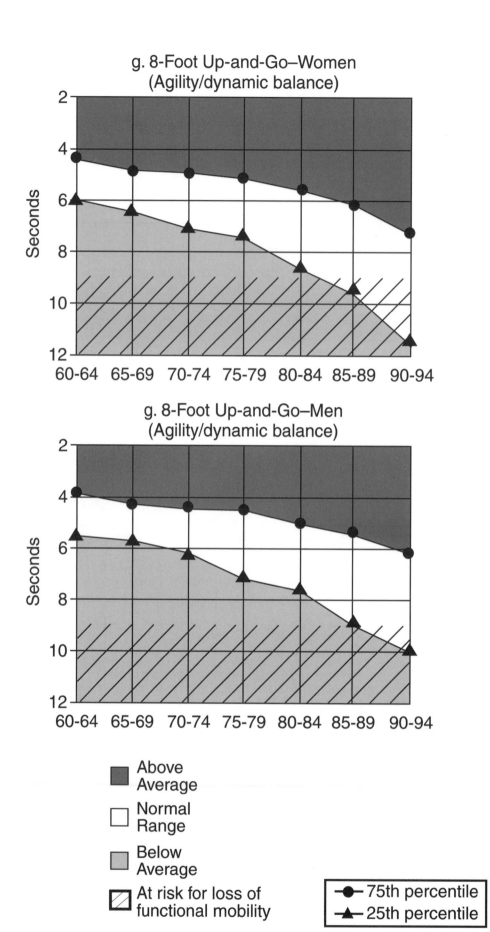

g. 8-Foot Up-and-Go–Women
(Agility/dynamic balance)

g. 8-Foot Up-and-Go–Men
(Agility/dynamic balance)

Above Average

Normal Range

Below Average

At risk for loss of functional mobility

75th percentile
25th percentile

Personal Goals/Activity Plans

Step 1. Describe at least one *long-term goal* you would like to achieve that could result from increased exercise. Goals can be specific, such as improving SFT walking scores from 500 to 600 yards in 6 minutes, or losing 10 pounds before a granddaughter's wedding next summer. Goals can be more general, such as increasing one's participation in moderate physical activity to the recommended 30-40 minutes per day on most days of the week.

Long-Term Goal or Major Exercise Objective: _____

Step 2. Describe realistic *short-term goals*, expressed as a two-week activity plan that will move you toward your goals. Be specific relative to your planned activities and a proposed schedule.

Activity	**Days/Times**
_____	_____
_____	_____
_____	_____
_____	_____
_____	_____

Step 3. Describe any potential obstacles that might keep you from following your plans and possible strategies for overcoming them.

Obstacle	**Strategy for Overcoming**
_____	_____
_____	_____
_____	_____
_____	_____
_____	_____

Step 4. Formalize your commitment to the above plan by signing on the line below. Discuss your plans with a friend, family member, or your exercise leader. Ask him or her to sign off as a witness and be willing to discuss your progress at least once a week.

Your Signature _____ Date _____

Witness Signature _____ Date _____

Activity Record

Week of _____

Name _____

Record # of minutes per day	Sunday	Monday	Tuesday	Wednesday	Thursday	Friday	Saturday
Lifestyle activity: Indicate any moderately strenuous housework, yard work, recreation, sports, etc. If low active, should add structured exercise (see below).							
Structured Exercise: *Aerobic exercise*—brisk walking, jogging, aerobic exercise, cycling, treadmill, etc. (Need 20-30 min 3-5 times a week.)							
Strengthening exercise—can use elastic band/tubing, hand weights, weight machines, or calisthenics. (Work upper and lower muscles at least 2 times a week.)							
Daily totals: Are you getting 30-40 min of moderate exercise on most days?							
Also important: *Flexibility/stretching*—should stretch all muscle/joint areas 2-3 times a week, preferrably daily.							
Agility/balance activities—especially important for those experiencing loss of balance.							

Appendix M

Normal Range of Scores for Women*

	60–64	65–69	70–74	75–79	80–84	85–89	90–94
Chair stand test (# of stands)	12-17	11-16	10-15	10-15	9-14	8-13	4-11
Arm curl test (# of reps)	13-19	12-18	12-17	11-17	10-16	10-15	8-13
6-minute walk test** (# of yd)	545-660	500-635	480-615	435-585	385-540	340-510	275-440
2-minute step test (# of steps)	75-107	73-107	68-101	68-100	60-90	55-85	44-72
Chair sit-and-reach test[†] (in. +/–)	–0.5-+5.0	–0.5-+4.5	–1.0-+4.0	–1.5-+3.5	–2.0-+3.0	–2.5-+2.5	–4.5-+1.0
Back scratch test[†] (in. +/–)	–3.0-+1.5	–3.5-+1.5	–4.0-+1.0	–5.0-+0.5	–5.5-+0.0	–7.0--1.0	–8.0--1.0
8-foot up-and-go test (sec)	6.0-4.4	6.4-4.8	7.1-4.9	7.4-5.2	8.7-5.7	9.6-6.2	11.5-7.3

Normal Range of Scores for Men*

	60–64	65–69	70–74	75–79	80–84	85–89	90–94
Chair stand test (# of stands)	14-19	12-18	12-17	11-17	10-15	8-14	7-12
Arm curl test (# of reps)	16-22	15-21	14-21	13-19	13-19	11-17	10-14
6-minute walk test** (# of yd)	610-735	560-700	545-680	470-640	445-605	380-570	305-500
2-minute step test (# of steps)	87-115	86-116	80-110	73-109	71-103	59-91	52-86
Chair sit-and-reach test[†] (in. +/–)	–2.5-+4.0	–3.0-+3.0	–3.0-+3.0	–4.0-+2.0	–5.5-+1.5	–5.5-+0.5	–6.5--0.5
Back scratch test[†] (in. +/–)	–6.5-+0.0	–7.5--1.0	–8.0--1.0	–9.0--2.0	–9.5--2.0	–9.5--3.0	–10.5--4.0
8-foot up-and-go test (sec)	5.6-3.8	5.9-4.3	6.2-4.4	7.2-4.6	7.6-5.2	8.9-5.5	10.0-6.2

* Normal range of scores is defined as the middle 50 percent of each age group. Scores above the range would be considered "above average" for the age group and those below the range would be "below average."

** Scores are rounded to the nearest five yards.

[†] Scores are rounded to the nearest half-inch.

Appendix N

Resources on Exercise Programming for Older Adults

Books

Allen, Lynn, Editor. 1999. *Active Older Adults.* Champaign, IL: Human Kinetics.

Clark, Janie. 1992. *Full Life Fitness: A Complete Exercise Program for Mature Adults.* Champaign, IL: Human Kinetics.

Cotton, Richard T., Editor. 1998. *Exercise for Older Adults: ACE's Guide for Fitness Professionals.* American Council on Exercise.

Evans, William and Irwin H. Rosenberg. 1991. *Biomarkers: The 10 Determinants of Aging You Can Control.* New York: Simon & Schuster.

National Institute on Aging, Baltimore. n.d. *Exercise: A Guide from the National Institute on Aging.* Publication No. NIH 98-4258.

Nelson, Miriam E. 1998. *Strong Women Stay Young.* New York: Bantam Books.

Osness, Wayne H., Editor. 1998. *Exercise and the Older Adult.* Dubuque, IA: Kendall/Hunt.

Van Norman, Kay A. 1995. *Exercise Programming for Older Adults.* Champaign, IL: Human Kinetics.

Wescott, W.L. and T.R. Baechle. 1999. *Strength Training for Seniors.* Champaign, IL: Human Kinetics.

Videos

Fitness Forever: The Exercise Program for Healthy Aging, featuring Nancy Swayzee, MES (Fitness Forever, 1998, 800-985-5185).

Movin' Out: Senior Style, featuring Laura Gladwin, MS (Peak Productions, 1991, 800-446-2322, ext. 414).

Sit and Be Fit, featuring Mary Ann Wilson, RN (Sit and Be Fit, 1991, 509-448-9438).

Web Sites

AAHPERD (American Alliance for Health, Physical Education, Recreation and Dance)—**www.aahperd.org**

ACE (American Council on Exercise)—**www.acefitness.com**

ACSM (American College of Sports Medicine)—**www.acsm.org**

AFAA (Aerobics & Fitness Association of America)—**www.afaa.com**

IDEA (International Dance Exercise Association)—**www.ideafit.com**

ISAPA (International Society for Aging and Physical Activity)—**www.isapa.org**

Keiser Institute on Aging—**www.keiserinstituteonaging.com**

50-Plus Fitness Association—**www.50plus.org**

The contact information included in this list was correct at the time of publication.

Appendix O

Measurement Conversions

To convert measurements from English to metric, use these conversion charts. Multiply the English measurement by the appropriate conversion factor using all the decimal places.

Weight

To change	To	Multiply by
pounds (lb)	kilograms (kg)	.453592

Length

To change	To	Multiply by
inches (in.)	centimeters (cm)	2.540005
feet (ft)	meters (m)	.3048006
yards (yd)	meters (m)	.91440183
miles (mi)	kilometers (Km)	1.60935

References

Ainsworth, B.E., Montoye, H.J., & Leon, A.S. (1994). Methods of assessing physical activity during leisure and work. In C. Bouchard, R.J. Shephard, & T. Stephens (Eds.), *Physical activity, fitness, and health* (pp. 146-159). Champaign, IL: Human Kinetics.

Alexander, N.B., Schultz, A.B., & Warwick, D.N. (1991). Rising from a chair: Effects of age and functional ability on performance biomechanics. *Journal of Gerontology: Medical Sciences, 46,* M91-M98.

Alliance for Aging Research. (1999). *Independence for older Americans: An investment for our nation's future.* Washington, DC: Alliance for Aging Research.

American Academy of Orthopaedic Surgeons. (1966). *Joint motion: Method of measuring and recording.* Edinburgh: Livingstone.

American College of Sports Medicine. (1991). *Guidelines for exercise testing and prescription* (4th ed.). Philadelphia: Lea and Febiger.

American College of Sports Medicine. (1995). *Guidelines for exercise testing and prescription.* Philadelphia: Lippincott Williams & Wilkins.

American College of Sports Medicine. (1997). *Exercise management for persons with chronic diseases and disabilities.* Champaign, IL: Human Kinetics.

American College of Sports Medicine. (1998a). ACSM Position Stand on Exercise and Physical Activity for Older Adults. *Medicine and Science in Sports and Exercise, 30,* 992-1008.

American College of Sports Medicine. (1998b). *ACSM's resource manual for guidelines for exercise testing and prescription.* Philadelphia: Lippincott Williams & Wilkins.

American College of Sports Medicine. (2000). *Guidelines for exercise testing and prescription.* (6th edition.) Philadelphia: Lippincott Williams & Wilkins.

American Psychological Association. (1985). *Standards for educational and psychological tests.* Washington, DC: American Psychological Association.

Badley, E.M., Wagstaff, S., & Wood, P.H.N. (1984). Measures of functional ability (disability) in arthritis in relation to impairment of range of joint movement. *Annals of Rheumatic Disease, 43,* 563-569.

Baumgartner, T.A., & Jackson, A.S. (1999). *Measurement for evaluation in physical education and exercise science* (6th ed.). Boston: McGraw-Hill.

Bell, R.D., Hoshizaki, B., & Collins, M.L. (1983). *The post 50 "3-S" physical performance test.* Victoria, BC: R.E. & P. Holdings.

Bittner, V., Weiner, D.H., Yusuf, S., Rogers, W.J., McIntyre, K.M., Bangdiwala, S.I., Kronenberg, M.W., Kostis, J.B., Kohn, R.M., Guillotte, M., Greenberg, B., Woods, P.A., & Bourassa, M.G. (1993). Prediction of mortality and morbidity with a

6-minute walk test in patients with left ventricular dysfunction. *Journal of the American Medical Association, 270,* 1702-1707.

Bohannon, R.W. (1995). Sit-to-stand test for measuring performance of lower extremity muscles. *Perceptual and Motor Skills, 80,* 163-166.

Booth, F.W., Gordon, S.E., Carlson, C.J., & Hamilton, M.T. (2000). Waging war on modern chronic diseases: Primary prevention through exercise biology. *Journal of Applied Physiology, 88,* 774-787.

Borg, G. (1998). *Borg's perceived exertion and pain scales.*

Bouchard, C., Shephard, R.J., & Stephens, T. (1994). *Physical activity, fitness, and health.* Champaign, IL: Human Kinetics.

Boyd, M., & Zizzi, M. (1999). Strength, functional gains, and wellness perception in healthy older adults participating in the Vigor Weight Training Program. *Journal of Aging and Physical Activity, 7,* 299-330.

Bravo, G., Gauthier, P., Roy, P., Tessier, D., Gaulin, P., Dubois, M., & Peloquin, L. (1994). The functional fitness assessment battery: Reliability and validity data for elderly women. *Journal of Aging and Physical Activity, 2,* 67-79.

Brouha, L. (1943). A step test: A simple method of measuring physical fitness for muscular work in young men. *Research Quarterly, 14,* 31-36.

Brown, M., Sinacore, D.R., & Host, H.H. (1995). The relationship of strength to function in the older adult. *Journal of Gerontology, 50A* (Special Issue), 55-59.

Buchner, D.M. (1995). Clinical assessment of physical activity in older adults. In L.Z. Rubenstein, D. Wieland, & R. Bernabei (Eds.), *Geriatric assessment technology: The state of the art* (pp. 147-159). Milano: Editrice Kurtis.

Buchner, D.M., Guralnik, J.M., & Cress, M.E. (1995). The clinical assessment of gait, balance, and mobility in older adults. In L.Z. Rubenstein, D. Wieland, & R. Bernabei (Eds.), *Geriatric assessment technology: The state of the art* (pp. 75-89). Milano: Editrice Kurtis.

Cailliet, R. (1988). *Low back pain syndrome.* Philadelphia: Davis.

Chakravarty, K., & Webley, M. (1993). Shoulder joint movement and its relationship to disability in the elderly. *Journal of Rheumatology, 20,* 1359-1361.

Chandler, J.M., & Hadley, E.C. (1996). Exercise to improve physiologic and functional performance in old age. *Clinics in Geriatric Medicine, 12,* 761-784.

Cooper Institute for Aerobics Research. (1999). *The Fitnessgram test administration manual* (2nd ed.). Champaign, IL: Human Kinetics.

Cooper, K.H. (1968). A means of assessing maximal oxygen intake. *Journal of the American Medical Association, 203,* 135-138.

Cooper, K.H. (1995). Anything that I may do for you? Keynote presentation at annual conference of the American Alliance for Health, Physical Education, Recreation and Dance. Portland, OR.

Cotten, D.J. (1971). A modified step test for group cardiovascular testing. *Research Quarterly, 42,* 91-95.

Cress, M.E., Buchner, D.M., Questad, K.A., Esselman, P.C., deLateur, B.J., & Schwartz, R.S. (1996). Continuous-scale physical functional performance in a broad range of older adults. *Archives and Physical Medicine and Rehabilitation, 77,* 1243-1250.

Cress, M.E., Thomas, D.P., Johnson, J., Kasch, F.W., Cassens, R.G., Smith, E.L., & Agre, J.C. (1991). Effect of training on $\dot{V}O_2$max, thigh strength, and muscle morphology in septuagenarian women. *Medicine and Science in Sport and Exercise, 23,* 752-758.

Csuka, M., & McCarty, D.J. (1985). Simple method for measurement of lower extremity muscle strength. *American Journal of Medicine, 78,* 77-81.

DiPietro, L. (1996). The epidemiology of physical activity and physical function in older people. *Medicine and Science in Sports and Exercise, 28,* 596-600.

Disch, J., Frankiewicz, R., & Jackson, A. (1975). Construct validation of distance run tests. *Research Quarterly, 46,* 169-176.

Dugas, E.W. (1996). *The development and validation of a 2-minute step test to estimate aerobic endurance in older adults.* Unpublished master's thesis, California State University, Fullerton.

Evans, W., & Rosenberg, I.H. (1991). *Biomarkers: The 10 determinants of aging you can control.* New York: Simon & Schuster.

Evans, W.J. (1995). Effects of exercise on body composition and functional capacity of the elderly. *Journal of Gerontology, 50A,* 147-150.

Fenstermaker, K.L., Plowman, S.A., & Looney, M.A. (1992). Validation of the Rockport Fitness Walking Test in females 65 years and older. *Research Quarterly for Exercise and Sport, 63,* 322-327.

Fiatarone, M.A., & Evans, W.J. (1993). The etiology and reversibility of muscle dysfunction in the aged. *Journal of Gerontology, 44,* 77-83.

Fiatarone, M.A., Marks, E.C., Ryan, N.D., Meredith, C.N., Lipsitz, L.A., & Evans, W.J. (1990). High-intensity strength training in nonagenarians: Effects on skeletal muscle. *Journal of the American Medical Association, 263,* 3029-3034.

Fiatarone, M.A., O'Neill, E.F., Ryan, N.D., Clements, K.M., Solares, G.R., Nelson, M.E., Roberts, S.B., Kehayias, J.J., Lipsitz, L.A., & Evans, W.J. (1994). Exercise training and nutritional supplementation for physical frailty in very elderly people. *New England Journal of Medicine, 330,* 1769-1775.

Fried, L.P., Ettinger, W.H., Lind, B., Newman, A.B., & Gardin, J. (1994). Physical disability in older adults: A physiological approach. *Journal of Clinical Epidemiology, 47,* 747-760.

Galanos, A.N., Peiper, C.F., Cornoni-Huntley, J., Bales, C.W., & Fillenbaum, G.G. (1994). Nutrition and function: Is there a relationship between body mass index and the functional capabilities of community dwelling elderly? *Journal of the American Geriatric Society, 42,* 368-373.

Gill, T.M., Williams, C.S., Richardson, E.D., & Tinetti, M.E. (1996). Impairments in physical performance and cognitive status as predisposing factors for functional dependence among nondisabled older persons. *Journal of Gerontology: Medical Sciences, 51A,* M283-M288.

Gill, T.M., Williams, C.S., & Tinetti, M.E. (1995). Assessing risk for the onset of functional dependence among older adults: The role of physical performance. *Journal of the American Geriatric Society, 43,* 603-609.

Golding, L., Myers, C., & Sinning, W. (1989). *Y's way to physical fitness* (3rd ed.). Champaign, IL: Human Kinetics.

Grabiner, M.K., Koh, T.J., Lundin, T.M., & Jahnigen, D.W. (1993). Kinematics of recovery from a stumble. *Journal of Gerontology, 48,* M97-M102.

Gross, J., Fetto, J., & Rosen, E. (1996). *Musculoskeletal examination.* Cambridge: Blackwell Science.

Guralnik, J.M., Ferrucci, L., Simonsick, E.M., Salive, M.E., & Wallace, R.B. (1995). Lower-extremity function in persons over the age of 70 years as a predictor of subsequent disability. *New England Journal of Medicine, 332,* 556-561.

Guralnik, J.M., Simonsick, E.M., Ferrucci, L., Glynn, R.J., Berkman, L.F., Blazer, D.G., Scherr, P.A., & Wallace, R.B. (1994). A short physical performance battery assessing lower extremity function: Association with self-reported disability and prediction of mortality and nursing home admission. *Journal of Gerontology, 49,* M85-M94.

Guyatt, G.H., Sullivan, M.J., Thompson, P.J., Fallen, E.I., Pugsley, S.O., Taylor, D.W., & Berman, L.B. (1985a). The 6-minute walk: A new measure of exercise capacity in patients with chronic heart failure. *Canadian Medical Association Journal, 132,* 919-923.

Guyatt, G.H., Thompson, P.J., Berman, L.B., Sullivan, M.J., Townsend, M., Jones, N.L., & Pugsley, S.O. (1985b). How should we measure function in patients with chronic heart and lung disease. *Journal of Chronic Disabilities, 38,* 517-524.

Hagberg, J., Graves, J., Limacher, M., Woods, D., Cononie, C., Leggett, S., Gruber, J., & Pollock, M. (1989). Cardiovascular responses of 70-79 year old men and women to exercise training. *Journal of Applied Physiology, 66,* 2589-2594.

Hagberg, J.M. (1994). Physical activity, fitness, health, and aging. In C. Bouchard, R. Shephard, & T. Stephens (Eds.), *Physical activity, fitness, and health: International proceedings and consensus statement* (pp. 993-1005). Champaign, IL: Human Kinetics.

Harris, T., Kovar, M.G., Suzman, R., Kleinman, J.C., & Feldman, J.J. (1989). Longitudinal study of physical ability in the oldest-old. *American Journal of Public Health, 79,* 698-702.

Haskell, W.L., & Phillips, W.T. (1995). Exercise training, fitness, health, and longevity. In D.L. Lamb, C.V. Gisolfi, & E. Nadel (Eds.), *Perspectives in exercise and sports medicine: Exercise in older adults* (Vol. 8, pp. 11-52). Carmel, IN: Cooper.

Hoppenfeld, S. (1976). *Physical examination of the spine and extremities.* Norwalk, CT: Appleton & Lange.

Hubert, H.B., Bloch, D.A., & Fries, J.F. (1993). Risk factors for physical disability in an aging cohort: The NHANES I epidemiologic followup study. *Journal of Rheumatology, 20,* 480-488.

Hubley-Kozey, C.L., Wall, J.C., & Hogan, D.B. (1995). Effects of a general exercise program on passive hip, knee, and ankle range of motion of older women. *Topics in Geriatric Rehabilitation, 10,* 33-44.

Hurley, B.F., & Hagberg, J.M. (1998). Optimizing health in older persons: Aerobic or strength training? In J. Holloszy (Ed.), *Exercise and sport science reviews* (Vol. 26, pp. 61-89). Baltimore: Williams & Wilkins.

Jackson, A.S., Beard, E.F., Wier, L.T., Ross, R.M., Stuteville, J.E., & Blair, S.N. (1995). Changes in aerobic power of men, ages 25-70 years. *Medicine and Science in Sports and Exercise, 27,* 113-120.

Jackson, A.S., Wier, L.T., Ayers, G.W., Beard, E.F., Stuteville, J.E., & Blair, S.N. (1996). Changes in aerobic power of women, ages 20-64 yr. *Medicine and Science in Sports and Exercise, 28,* 884-891.

Jackson, A.W., & Baker, A.A. (1986). The relationship of the sit and reach test to criterion measures of hamstring and back flexibility in young females. *Research Quarterly for Exercise and Sport, 57,* 183-186.

Jackson, A.W., & Langford, N.J. (1989). The criterion-related validity of the sit-and-reach test: Replication and extension of previous findings. *Research Quarterly for Exercise and Sport, 60,* 384-387.

James, T.W. (1999). *The 30-second arm curl test as an indicator of upper body strength in older adults.* Unpublished master's thesis, California State University, Fullerton.

Johnston, J. (1999). *Validation of a 2-minute step-in-place test relative to treadmill performance in older adults.* Unpublished master's thesis, California State University, Fullerton.

Jones, C.J., & Rikli, R.E. (1999). Physical decline in older adults as a function of age, gender, and physical activity level. *Medicine and Science in Sports and Exercise, 31,* S379.

Jones, C.J., Rikli, R.E., & Beam, W.C. (1999). A 30-s chair-stand test as a measure of lower body strength in community-residing older adults. *Research Quarterly for Exercise and Sport, 70,* 113-119.

Jones, C.J., Rikli, R.E., Max, J., & Noffal, G. (1998). The reliability and validity of a chair sit-and-reach test as a measure of hamstring flexibility in older adults. *Research Quarterly for Exercise and Sport, 69,* 338-343.

Judge, J.O. (1993). Functional importance of muscular strength. *Topics in Geriatric Rehabilitation, 8,* 38-50.

Kaplan, G.A., Strawbridge, W.J., Camacho, T., & Cohen, R.D. (1993). Factors associated with change in physical functioning in the elderly: A six-year prospective study. *Journal of Aging and Health, 5,* 140-153.

Kendall, F.P., McCreary, E.K., & Provance, P.G. (1993). *Muscles: Testing and function* (4th ed.). Baltimore: Williams & Wilkins.

Kline, G.M., Porcari, J.P., Hintermeister, R., Freedson, P.S., Ward, A., McCarron, R.F., Ross, J., & Rippe, J.M. (1987). Estimation of $\dot{V}O_2$max from a one-mile track walk, gender, age, and body weight. *Medicine and Science in Sports and Exercise, 19,* 253-259.

Kohrt, W., Malley, M., Goggan, A., Spina, R., Ogawa, T., Ehsani, A., Bourey, R., Martin, W., & Holloszy, J. (1991). Effects of gender, age, and fitness level on response of $\dot{V}O_2$max to training in 60-71 yr olds. *Journal of Applied Physiology, 71,* 2004-2011.

Konczak, J., Meeuwsen, H.J., & Cress, M.E. (1992). Changing affordances in stair climbing: The perception of maximum climbability in young and old adults. *Journal of Experimental Psychology: Human Perception and Performance, 18,* 691-697.

Lacroix, A.Z., Guralnik, J.M., Berkman, L.F., Wallace, R.B., & Satterfield, S. (1993). Maintaining mobility in late life II: Smoking, alcohol consumption, physical activity, and body mass index. *American Journal of Epidemiology, 137,* 858-869.

Lawrence, R., & Jette, A.M. (1996). Disentangling the disablement process. *Journal of Gerontology: Social Sciences, 51B,* 5173-5182.

Liemohn, W., Snodgrass, L.B., & Sharpe, G.L. (1988). Unresolved controversies in back management—A review. *Journal of Orthopaedic and Sports Physical Therapy, 9,* 239-244.

Losonczy, K.G., Harris, T.B., Cornoni-Huntley, J., Simonsick, E.M., Wallace, R.B., Cook, N.R., Ostfeld, A.M., & Blazer, D.G. (1995). Does weight loss from middle age to old age explain the inverse weight mortality relation in old age? *American Journal of Epidemiology, 141,* 312-321.

MacRae, P., Feltner, M., & Reinsch, S. (1994). A 1-year exercise program for older women: Effects on falls, injuries, and physical performance. *Journal of Aging and Physical Activity, 2,* 127-142.

MacRae, P.G., Lacourse, M., & Moldavon, R. (1992). Physical performance measures that predict faller status in community-dwelling older adults. *Journal of Occupational and Sports Physical Therapy, 16*, 123-128.

Magee, D.J. (1992). *Orthopedic physical assessment.* Philadelphia: W.B. Saunders.

McArdle, W.D., Katch, F.I., Pechar, G.S., Jacobson, L., & Ruck, S. (1972). Reliability and interrelationships between maximal oxygen intake, physical work capacity and step-test scores in college women. *Medicine and Science in Sports, 4*, 182-186.

McCartney, N., Hicks, A.L., Martin, J., & Webber, C. (1996). A longitudinal trial of weight training in the elderly: Continued improvements in year 2. *Journal of Gerontology, 51*(B).

McMurdo, M.E., & Rennie, L. (1993). A controlled trial of exercise by residents of old people's homes. *Age and Aging, 22*, 11-15.

Miotto, J.M., Chodzko-Zajko, W.J., Reich, J.L., & Supler, M.M. (1999). Reliability and validity of the Fullerton Functional Fitness Test: An independent replication study. *Journal of Aging and Physical Activity, 7*, 339-353.

Morey, M.C., Cowper, P.A., Feussner, J.R., Dipasquale, R.C., Crowley, G.M., & Sullivan, R.J. (1991). Two-year trends in physical performance following supervised exercise among community-dwelling old veterans. *Journal of the American Geriatric Society, 38*, 549-554.

Morey, M.C., Pieper, C.F., & Cornoni-Huntley, J. (1998). Physical fitness and functional limitations in community-dwelling older adults. *Medicine and Science in Sports and Exercise, 30*, 715-723.

Nagi, S.Z. (1965). Some conceptual issues in disability and rehabilitation. In M.B. Sussman (Ed.), *Sociology and rehabilitation* (pp. 100-113). Washington, DC: American Sociological Association.

Nagi, S.Z. (1991). Disability concepts revisited: Implication for prevention. In A.M. Pope & A.R. Tarlov (Eds.), *Disability in America: Toward a national agenda for prevention* (pp. 309-327). Washington, DC: National Academy Press.

Nelson, M., Fiatarone, M., Morganti, C., Trice, E., Greenberg, R., & Evans, W. (1994). Effects of high-intensity strength training on multiple risk factors for osteoporotic fractures. *Journal of the American Medical Association, 272*, 1909-1914.

Nichols, J.F., Hitzelberger, L.M., Sherman, J.G., & Patterson, P. (1995). Effects of resistance training on muscular strength and functional abilities of community-dwelling older adults. *Journal of Aging and Physical Activity, 3*, 238-250.

Osness, W.H., Adrian, M., Clark, B., Hoeger, W., Rabb, D., & Wiswell, R. (1996). *Functional fitness assessment for adults over 60 years.* Dubuque, IA: Kendall/Hunt.

Paffenbarger, R.S.J., Blair, S.N., Lee, I.M., & Hyde, R.T. (1993). Measurement of physical activity to assess health effects in free-living populations. *Medicine and Science in Sports and Exercise, 25*, 60-70.

Paterson, D.H., Cunningham, D.A., Koval, J.J., & St. Croix, C.M. (1999). Aerobic fitness in a population of independently living men and women ages 55-86 years. *Medicine & Science in Sports & Exercise, 21*, 1813-1820.

Patterson, P., Wiksten, D.L., Ray, L., Flanders, C., & Sanphy, D. (1996). The validity and reliability of the back saver sit-and-reach test in middle school girls and boys. *Research Quarterly for Exercise and Sport, 64*, 448-451.

Peloquin, L., Gauthier, P., Bravo, G., Lacombe, G., & Billiard, J. (1998). Reliability and validity of the 5-minute walking field test for estimating $\dot{V}O_2$ peak in elderly subjects with knee osteoarthritis. *Journal of Aging and Physical Activity, 6*, 36-44.

Pendergast, D.R., Fisher, N.M., & Calkins, E. (1993). Cardiovascular, neuromuscular, and metabolic alterations with age leading to frailty. *Journal of Gerontology, 48* (Special Issue), 61-67.

Podsiadlo, D., & Richardson, S. (1991). The timed "up and go": A test of basic functional mobility for frail elderly persons. *Journal of the American Geriatric Society, 39*, 142-148.

Province, M.A., Hadley, E.C., Hornbrook, M.C., Lipsitz, L.A., Miller, J.P., Mulrow, C.D., Ory, M.G., Sattin, R.W., Tinetti, M.E., & Wolf, S.L. (1995). The effects of exercise on falls in elderly patients. A pre-planned meta-analysis of the FICSIT trials. *Journal of the American Medical Association, 273*, 1341-1347.

Pyka, G., Lindenberger, E., Charette, S., & Marcus, R. (1994). Muscle strength and fiber adaptations to a year-long resistance training program in elderly men and women. *Journal of Gerontology, 49*, M22-M27.

Rakowski, W., & Mor, V. (1992). The association of physical activity with mortality among older adults in the longitudinal study of aging (1984-1988). *Journal of Gerontology, 47*, M122-M129.

Rikli, R.E., & Edwards, D. (1991). Effects of a three-year exercise program on motor function and cognitive processing speed in older women. *Research Quarterly for Exercise and Sport, 62*, 61-67.

Rikli, R.E., & Jones, C.J. (1997). Assessing physical performance in independent older adults: Issues and guidelines. *Journal of Aging and Physical Activity, 5*, 244-261.

Rikli, R.E., & Jones, C.J. (1998). The reliability and validity of a 6-minute walk test as a measure of physical endurance in older adults. *Journal of Aging and Physical Activity, 6*, 363-375.

Rikli, R.E., & Jones, C.J. (1999a). Development and validation of a functional fitness test for community-residing older adults. *Journal of Aging and Physical Activity, 7*, 127-159.

Rikli, R.E., & Jones, C.J. (1999b). Functional fitness normative scores for community-residing adults, ages 60-94. *Journal of Aging and Physical Activity, 7*, 160-179.

Rikli, R.E., & Jones, C.J. (2000). Physical activity level, fitness, and functional ability of community-residing older adults. *Medicine and Science in Sports and Exercise, 32*, 218.

Rikli, R.E., Jones, C.J., Beam, W.B., Duncan, S.J., & Lamar, B. (1996). Testing versus training effects on 1RM strength measures in older adults. *Medicine and Science in Sports and Exercise, 28*, S153.

Rose, D.J., Jones, C.J., Dickin, C., Lemon, N., & Bories, T. (1999). The effect of a community-based balance and mobility training program on functional performance and balance-related self-confidence in older adults with a history of falls. *Journal of Aging and Physical Activity, 7*, 265-266.

Safrit, M.J., & Wood, T.M. (1995). *Introduction to measurement in physical education and exercise science.* St. Louis: Mosby-Year Book.

Schoenfeld, D.E., Malmrose, L.C., Blazer, D.G., Gold, D.T., & Seeman, T.E. (1994). Self-rated health and mortality in the high-functioning elderly—A closer look at healthy individuals: MacArthur field study of successful aging. *Journal of Gerontology, 49*, M109-M115.

Schroeder, J. (1995). A comprehensive survey of older adult exercise programs in two California communities. *Journal of Aging and Physical Activity, 3*, 290-298.

Seeman, T.E., Berkman, L.F., Charpentier, P.A., Blazer, D.G., Alpert, M.A., & Tinetti, M.E. (1995). Behavioral and psychosocial predictors of physical performance: MacArthur Studies of Successful Aging. *Journal of Gerontology, 50*, M177-M183.

Seeman, T.E., Charpentier, P.A., Berkman, L.F., Tinetti, M.E., Guralnik, J.M., Albert, M., Blazer, D., & Rowe, J.W. (1994). Predicting changes in physical performance in a high-functioning elderly cohort: MacArthur Studies of Successful Aging. *Journal of Gerontology, 49*, M97-M108.

Select Committee on Aging, U. S. House of Representatives. (1992). *Aging research: Benefits outweigh the costs* (Publication No. 102-871). Washington, DC: U.S. Government Printing Office.

Shephard, R.J. (1997). *Aging, physical activity, and health.* Champaign, IL: Human Kinetics.

Simonsick, E.M., Lafferty, M.E., Phillips, C.L., Mendes de Leon, C.F., Kasl, S.V., Seeman, T.E., Fillenbaum, G., Hebert, P., & Lemke, J.H. (1993). Risk due to inactivity in physically capable older adults. *American Journal of Public Health, 83*, 1443-1450.

Sperling, L. (1980). Evaluation of upper extremity function in 70-year-old men and women. *Scandinavian Journal of Rehabilitative Medicine, 12*, 139-144.

Spirduso, W.W. (1995). *Physical dimensions of aging.* Champaign, IL: Human Kinetics.

Starkey, C., & Ryan, J.L. (1996). *Evaluation of orthopedic and athletic injuries.* Philadelphia: Davis.

Steele, B. (1996). Timed walking tests of exercise capacity in chronic cardiopulmonary illness. *Journal of Cardiopulmonary Rehabilitation, 16*, 25-33.

Stewart, A.L., Hays, R.D., Wells, K.B., Rogers, W.H., Spritzer, K.L., & Greenfield, S. (1994). Long-term functioning and well-being outcomes associated with physical activity and exercise in patients with chronic conditions in the Medical Outcomes Study. *Journal of Clinical Epidemiology, 47*, 719-730.

Stump, T., Clark, D.O., Johnson, R.J., & Wolinsky, F.D. (1997). The structure of health status among Hispanic, African American, and White older adults. *The Journals of Gerontology, 52B* (Special Issue), 49-60.

Tinetti, M.E., Speechley, M., & Ginter, S.F. (1988). Risk factors for falls among elderly persons living in the community. *New England Journal of Medicine, 319*, 1701-1707.

Tinetti, M.E., Williams, T.F., & Mayewski, R. (1986). Fall risk index for elderly patients based on number of chronic conditions. *American Journal of Medicine, 80*, 429-434.

U.S. Bureau of the Census. (1996). *Sixty-five plus in the United States: Current population reports* (P23-190). Washington, DC: U.S. Department of Commerce.

U.S. Department of Health and Human Services. (1990). *Healthy People 2000: National health promotion and disease prevention objectives* (PHS 91-50213). Washington, DC: U.S. Government Printing Office.

U.S. Department of Health and Human Services. (1991). *Physical frailty: A reducible barrier to independence for older Americans.* (NIH91-397). Washington, DC: U.S. Government Printing Office.

U.S. Department of Health and Human Services. (1996). *Physical activity and health: A report of the surgeon general.* Atlanta: U.S. Department of Health and Human

Services, Centers for Disease Control and Prevention, National Center for Chronic Disease Prevention and Health Promotion.

U.S. Department of Health and Human Services. (1999). *Healthy People 2000 Review, 1998-99* (PHS 99-1256). Washington, DC: U.S. Government Printing Office.

U.S. Department of Housing and Urban Development. (1999). *Housing our elders.* Washington, DC: Office of Policy Development and Research.

Verfaillie, D.F., Nichols, J.F., Turkel, E., & Hovell, M.F. (1997). Effects of resistance, balance, and gait training on reduction of risk factors leading to falls in elders. *Journal of Aging and Physical Activity, 5,* 213-228.

Warren, B.J., Dotson, R.G., Nieman, D.C., & Butterworth, D.E. (1993). Validation of a 1-mile walk test in elderly women. *Journal of Aging and Physical Activity, 1,* 13-21.

Winnick, J.P., & Short, F.X. (1999). *The Brockport physical fitness test manual.* Champaign, IL: Human Kinetics.

INDEX

Note: The italicized *f* and *t* following page numbers refers to figures and tables, respectively.

About the Authors

Roberta E. Rikli, PhD, is professor and chair of the division of kinesiology and health promotion at California State University in Fullerton and is cofounder of the LifeSpan Wellness Program at Fullerton.

For the past 20 years, Dr. Rikli has done extensive work in physical performance assessment with a particular focus on senior fitness. She has published numerous scientific papers on her work and has made over 100 presentations at conferences and workshops in the United States, Germany, France, Finland, China, and Japan. She serves on the editorial boards of three scientific journals and is a regular reviewer for several others.

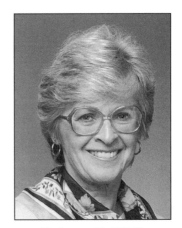

Roberta E. Rikli

She holds professional memberships in numerous organizations including the International Society for Aging and Physical Activity; the American Alliance for Health, Physical Education, Recreation and Dance (AAHPERD); the American College of Sports Medicine (ACSM); and the American Academy for Kinesiology and Physical Education.

Dr. Rikli lives in Orange, California, and enjoys hiking and playing tennis and golf.

C. Jessie Jones, PhD, is a professor of the division of kinesiology and health promotion at California State University in Fullerton and is codirector of the Center for Successful Aging at Fullerton.

Dr. Jones is internationally known for her research, program design, curriculum development, and instructor training in the field of exercise science and aging. She has taught senior fitness classes and conducted training workshops for senior fitness instructors for

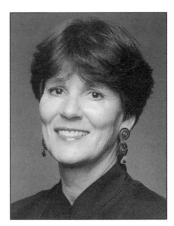

C. Jessie Jones

over 15 years. Her work has been covered in numerous publications and presented at conferences worldwide.

Her professional memberships include the Gerontological Society of America; the California Council for Gerontology and Geriatrics; the American Alliance for Health, Physical Education, Recreation and Dance (AAHPERD); and the American College of Sports Medicine (ACSM).

Dr. Jones also lives in Orange, California, where she enjoys hiking, playing golf, and dancing.

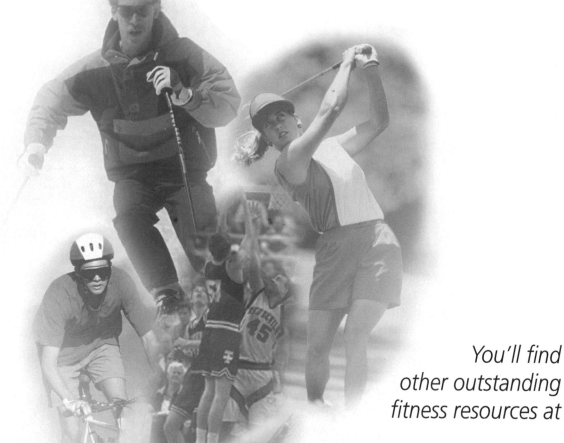

*You'll find
other outstanding
fitness resources at*

www.humankinetics.com

In the U.S. call

1-800-747-4457

Australia 08 8277 1555
Canada 1-800-465-7301
Europe .... +44 (0) 113 278 1708
New Zealand 09-523-3462

HUMAN KINETICS
The Information Leader in Physical Activity
P.O. Box 5076 • Champaign, IL 61825-5076 USA